ADDITIONA

THE PEANUT A

"*The Peanut Allergy Epidemic* is a masterful piece of medical detective work. Fraser has succeeded in doing what numerous specialists have proven unable to do—she has uncovered the cause of this iatrogenic phenomenon and given us an elegant explanation for why and how peanut allergy/anaphylaxis has emerged as a modern-day epidemic. With meticulous and thorough research and documentation, she explores and discredits the various theories that have been proposed as explanations for the rise in peanut allergy sufferers. . . . [It] is a vital, groundbreaking book, covering material that resides at the intersection of medicine, history, and public policy. I believe it should be required reading for everyone who administers injections, everyone who receives injections, and everyone who authorizes injections for children."

—Janet Levatin, board-certified pediatrician,
clinical instructor in pediatrics, Harvard Medical School

"Phenomenal detective work! Heather Fraser weaves history, medicine, and science into a convincing hypothesis to solve a modern medical mystery. *The Peanut Allergy Epidemic* explains the origins and recent dramatic rise in incidences of peanut allergy in particular, but also provides a context for a wide range of other increasingly common immunological diseases. It should be required reading for pediatricians. I hope it is read by parents and prospective parents everywhere before blindly consenting to prophylactic medical interventions for their children."

—Jamie Deckoff-Jones, MD

"I grew up on a diet of peanut butter and jelly sandwiches, which are now seen more as dangerous and scary toxins than comfort food. Yet amidst all the attention that has been brought to this mysterious rise of allergy, anaphylaxis, and even death (not to mention the highly profitable industry for remedies), no one in public health leadership has pointed to vaccines as a cause; this despite the fact that the word "allergy" was coined to describe reactions to injections. Fraser's book shows that the sudden change/increase in anaphylaxis in children coincided with the increase in childhood vaccination schedule, as well as the greater potency and increasing coverage rates for vaccines starting in the late 1980s through early 1990s. This rise in life-threatening reactions to peanuts, like other modern plagues like autism, was the beginning of what has become a widespread and epidemic. How long can we continue to hide our heads in the sand?"

—Mark Blaxill, Cofounder, Health Choice and the Canary Party,
coauthor, *The Age of Autism*

"As it tends to be with many autoimmune epidemics, more than one road leads to the development of the peanut allergy. It's Heather Fraser who makes a convincing argument that the four-way intersection of Newborn General Consent for Treatment, novel pharmaceutical frontiers, public health policy goals, and immunization administration convenience, paved the way for the high-speed anaphylactic expressway that is our "new normal" today. In a world where scientific research demands thorough investigation into all causes of the allergy epidemic but one, Heather Fraser stands alone, shining her light on the stones intentionally left unturned for the last quarter of a century."

—Robyn Ross, BS, JD, allergy advocate

"When we forget the history, we are bound to repeat it. In her book *The Peanut Allergy Epidemic*, Heather Fraser unravels the forgotten history of food allergy. She masterfully demonstrates how, time and again, bizarre appearances and wanings of widespread allergies to certain foods in human populations has followed the introduction and then withdrawal of specific medical formulations delivered by injection. Prior mass occurrences of allergy to specific foods came and went, but a modern epidemic of deadly peanut allergy is still expanding. Are we to accept this epidemic without asking why it is happening? Or should we strive to recognize the immunological cause so that the epidemic can be halted? The history of clinical and immunological research illuminated by *The Peanut Allergy Epidemic* paves the way to finding the cause that will first be vehemently denied, then ridiculed, and finally accepted."

—Tetyana Obukhanych, PhD, author, *Vaccine Illusion*

"Heather Fraser has written an important book that points to a false cost-benefit—in both economic and medical terms—in mass vaccinations. This is a compelling work on a subject that is taboo to the mainstream media."

—Lawrence Solomon, columnist, *Financial Post*,
and executive director of *Energy Probe*

"This magnificent book is in a rare class of books that present impeccable scientific evidence in prose that is accessible to the educated lay public, while slowly unfolding a gripping mystery that grabs the reader's attention all the way through. If Heather Fraser is right about the link between vaccines and peanut allergies, and the evidence speaks for itself, then it opens up the frightening possibility that vaccines play a major role in all the food allergies that beset today's children."

—Dr. Stephanie Seneff, senior research scientist,
MIT Computer Science and Artificial Intelligence Laboratory

"In a masterful account, historian Heather Fraser illuminates the statistics, theories, and politics of the peanut allergy epidemic, revealing intriguing parallels between this debacle and what other contemporary public health controversies, such as autism, face. This book is a must-read for anyone who wants to gain a broader perspective on the politics of public health."

—Teri Arranga, director of AutismOne,
editor in chief, *Autism Science Digest*

"*The Peanut Allergy Epidemic*, by Heather Fraser, is a book which has been eagerly anticipated by anyone dealing with food allergy, including parents, physicians, nurses, and teachers. Extensively researched and entertainingly written, the book contains a wealth of information about the history and the origins of the epidemic of the peanut allergy which has occurred in the past twenty years, as well as the vaccines and their additives that we have injected into our children in ever-increasing amounts over the same time period. It reads like a detective novel, but is all well documented and astonishingly true. This book should be required reading not only for parents and physicians dealing with a peanut allergy, but anyone connected to the vaccine industry or the Food and Drug Administration. Congratulations to Heather Fraser for having the courage to tell a story which will not be well received by the medical establishment, but needed to be told anyway."

—Roger A. Francis, MD, practicing physician in Nevada, Missouri,
and parent of Tony, age fifteen, with autism and a peanut allergy

"Why are children increasingly developing sometimes fatal allergies to peanuts? The answer may lie in Heather Fraser's well-written and well-researched book on the topic of childhood allergies, *The Peanut Allergy Epidemic*. Part mystery story, part scientific inquiry, Fraser's book should raise a lot of questions and open some previously closed minds."

—Christopher A. Shaw, PhD, professor, Department of Ophthalmology and Visual Sciences, University of British Columbia

THE
PEANUT ALLERGY EPIDEMIC

WHAT'S CAUSING IT AND HOW TO STOP IT

THIRD EDITION

HEATHER FRASER

FOREWORD BY ROBERT F. KENNEDY, JR.

PREFACE BY WOODROW FRASER-BOYCHUK

Skyhorse Publishing

Note: This book is not intended to replace any information provided by a physician.

For Woody, Daisy, and Rick

CONTENTS

Author's Note

"Only puny secrets need protection. Big discoveries are protected by public incredulity."

—*Marshall McLuhan*

Information is instant, constant, and exists all around us. This book is a product of the era of information and communication: an individual can find an answer to any question, if he is motivated.

I was motivated to write this book by an event for which I was completely unprepared. In 1995, my firstborn son at thirteen months of age had an anaphylactic reaction to peanut butter.

I wanted to know why.

Foreword

M y son Conor was born in 1994. He developed chronic asthma, food allergies, and anaphylaxis that required twenty-nine emergency room visits before he was three years old. His brother Finn, born four years later, also developed anaphylaxis. What were the chances? Neither their mother nor I had any allergies. I'm not even allergic to poison ivy!

Epidemic allergy in our children emerged suddenly, then ramped up inexorably, through the 1990s, in every American community. Its impacts affect our businesses, public spaces, transportation, and schools. Without explanation, children with severe allergies to peanuts, milk, fish, bee venom, latex, pollens, and more were filling our classrooms. Peanut allergy is now so prevalent that it impacts everyday consumer behavior; 30% of polled mothers said that nut allergy influenced a food purchase decision[1] and 67% considered nut allergy when buying snacks for an event with children.

We have all watched in bewilderment as peanut allergies among children skyrocketed from .8% in 2002 to 1.4% in 2008. Just three years later in 2011, another study indicated an incidence as high as 2.8%. Upwards of two million children in the United States are now allergic to peanuts. Schools learned to protect vulnerable kids with cupboards filled with EpiPens and puffers, hand-washing protocols, food bans and exempt spaces; inconveniences that sometimes annoy non-allergy families, but provided some reassurance to worried parents like me.

Initially, researchers believed peanut allergy was unique to western countries, specifically the United Kingdom, Canada, the United States, and Australia. Then, suddenly, similar epidemics exploded in Singapore, Hong Kong, and Africa. Where was this coming from? I knew the answer could not be solely genetic. As my friend, Dr. Boyd Haley, chairman emeritus of the University of

Kentucky Department of Chemistry, says, "Genes don't cause epidemics. Genes can provide the vulnerability, but you need an environmental toxin." But what toxin had launched the allergy cascade?

In 1998, I was among a group of New York parents who co-founded the Food Allergy Initiative (FAI) to research cures for food allergies. FAI did extraordinary work in developing treatments, but I remained intensely curious about identifying the cause. In my own research, I learned that a host of other childhood epidemics—autism, ADD, ADHD, SIDS, OCD, ASD, narcolepsy, sleep and seizure disorders, neurodevelopmental delays, autoimmune diseases, and tics—all began rising in the early 1990s. Coincidentally, this is the time period during which the Center for Disease Control and Prevention (CDC) dramatically expanded the vaccine schedule, raising children's exposure to mercury, aluminum, and other toxic vaccine ingredients. Public health authorities expanded the schedule, including the battery of metal-laden vaccines, first in the United States, the United Kingdom, and Canada—and subsequently in Asia and Africa—along a timeline exquisitely correlated with the explosion of these new childhood disease epidemics, in these locales.

Abundant peer-reviewed science linked mercury, a known neurotoxin, to the neurodevelopmental injuries that now, according to the CDC, afflict one in six American children. In 2013, I wrote a book assembling and synthesizing hundreds of these studies. As I searched the medical literature on PubMed, I occasionally came across studies linking these contaminants to anaphylaxis, asthma, allergies, and eczema. While the timing of the anaphylaxis explosion suggested a link to the sudden expansion of the vaccines schedule, the published science on its origins was surprisingly sparse.

Scientists and public health officials have offered numerous theories purporting to explain the epidemic: the hygiene hypothesis, GMOs, glyphosate-based pesticides, environmental pollutants, or peanut mold, for example. But the proliferations of these exposures did not neatly coincide with the allergy epidemics. None of these potential causes explained the sudden meteoric rise of anaphylaxis in the early 1990s.

Seeking answers that might help end the epidemic, the National Peanut Allergy Board, along with Food Allergy Research and Education (FARE) and the National Institutes of Health (NIH), funded the LEAP study (Learn Early About Peanut Allergy) in 2010. However, the study, which was published in 2015 in the *New England Journal of Medicine,* sheds little light on causation. We learned only that children at risk of developing peanut allergy were those who already had severe egg allergy and/or eczema. Serious allergy can lead to more allergies? That struck me as a circular conclusion; it brought us no closer to answering the riddle: What was triggering the cascade of allergy epidemics in the first place?

In the summer of 2016, I asked Dr. James Baker, head of the nonprofit FARE—formerly the FAI—and former senior vice president of Merck's vaccine division, whether vaccines could be a cause of the food allergy epidemic. He told me that it was a possibility that should be looked into. But, "unfortunately nobody is studying that at the moment." Dr. Baker's candor was refreshing. Most scientists understand the radioactive peril of raising questions that implicate vaccine safety. Scientists, like doctors and journalists, know that vaccine debate can be a career-ending minefield. For that reason, scientists interested in allergies tend to cluster around safe harbors like genetic studies or behavioral research. Funding is easier to find in these arenas, scientific journals are willing to publish such works and careers remain on trajectory. Unfortunately, such research has gotten us no closer to understanding the etiology of the epidemic.

Around the time of my discussion with Dr. Baker, I stumbled on Heather's book. I devoured it ravenously. Heather has done for allergies what Jared Diamond did for broader concepts of human history in his book, *Guns, Germs, and Steel*. Although she is not a scientist, she used her gift for synthesizing a wide range of scientific disciplines and history to arrive at a simple, coherent, integrated, and commonsense hypothesis that, for the first time, convincingly explains the sudden onset of the allergy epidemic. Her theory accounts for its steep rise in America in the early 1990s, and its subsequent movement from western nations into the developing world.

Heather tracks the allergy epidemic's causes to US political, legal, and medical reforms in the late 1980s. In 1986, the US National Childhood Vaccine Injury Act (NCVIA) and National Vaccine Injury Compensation Program (NVICP) eliminated liability for vaccine manufacturers; thereby creating a gold rush among vaccine makers. Any company shrewd or connected enough to persuade the CDC to add their products to the recommended schedule could cash in on the $30 billion vaccine bonanza. The vaccination schedule expanded rapidly without anybody performing comprehensive safety analyses or testing for possible negative synergies from the battery of multiple early immunizations. Nor did public health regulators make any effort to perform a mass loading calculation of the combined mercury and aluminum exposures, from so many new vaccines.

Having read Fraser's analysis, it seemed almost strange to me that no one had previously connected the dots between the greatly expanded vaccine schedule and the anaphylaxis crisis that preceded. Heather reveals how the answer to the anaphylaxis puzzle has always been buried in plain sight—in the accounts, detailed observations, and comments made by late nineteenth- and twentieth-century vaccine pioneers—concerning the tendency of vaccines to initiate anaphylaxis and allergy. Those pathbreaking vaccinologists had quickly discovered that injecting an allergen directly into the bloodstream, bypassing the digestive process, often provokes anaphylaxis. Medical literature shows how powerful adjuvants (most notably, aluminum), added to vaccines in order to increase the immunological response, also amplify the allergic response. Adjuvants promote allergic sensitization not just to vaccine antigens, but also to other "bystander" proteins and allergens in the ambient environment at the time that the adjuvanted vaccines were administered. Thus, a child vaccinated with aluminum adjuvants during a spring ragweed outbreak, may develop a lifelong allergy to ragweed. Similarly, a child immunized with a vaccine containing peanut oil, or similar proteins, may develop a deadly allergy to peanuts. Further, and as noted by the LEAP study, once a child has developed allergies there is a tendency to develop more.

It did not elude me that the same pharmaceutical companies that have transformed vaccination into a lucrative enterprise have also profited with additional billions on the back end, selling $600 EpiPens (two-pack), as well as puffers, nebulizers, steroids, Benadryl, and other medicines to injured children.

In August, 2016, I invited Heather to give a presentation to the Food Allergy Science Initiative (FASI) at the Broad Institute in Cambridge, Massachusetts. A prestigious group of well-funded and experienced scientists had gathered at MIT to find a way to "turn off" the allergic reaction by identifying genetic precursors to allergy. This is good and important work, but I wanted them to hear and understand Heather's story of the peanut allergy from a historical perspective, one that was supported by a rich library of medical literature. Using a series of vivid slides, Fraser clearly explained the provocative role of aluminum adjuvants, conjugate vaccine technology, and combination vaccines in the allergy explosion.

Fraser's presentation was strong and convincing, but it raised only mild interest among the scientists. They were not the least bit skeptical, but, they explained to us, "This is not what we do." Their expertise, they said, were human genes. When I questioned them, they acknowledged that the allergy epidemic must have been triggered by some environmental toxin, and that their research was unlikely to identify the culprit. They told me that they did not need to know what caused the peanut allergy in order to find a treatment. I began thinking that the refusal to look at the possible causal role of vaccines was like trying to find a genetic cause for sunburn without considering the role of the sun. Their work is important but while these scientists were trying to save the children downstream, I wanted to prevent a new generation of children from being pushed into the river in the first place. I believe that the reluctance among scientists to look at the role of vaccines is prolonging the epidemic and damaging the public's health.

Finally, for those of you who, like me, want to solve the food allergy mystery, Heather's book cracks the code.

Robert F. Kennedy, Jr.
President of Waterkeeper Alliance
Chairman of the World Mercury Project

Preface

"Peanut" has been a dirty word in my house for longer than I can remember; as if we were a family of wizards cowering in the shadow of Voldemort; as if by speaking the profanity we would bring down a mortal curse on our first-born son (myself). My mother can barely stand to imagine myself and a peanut in the same mental frame. It's no wonder; she's seen me on the brink of death four times (too many) and swollen like a balloon, with my dignity battered, after losing a duel with the dastardly plant. Of course, the taboo around the word has softened as I've grown older and more capable of self-defense, and am out of the home for most of the year. Even so, my mother's mind is still visibly set on edge if I tell her I've forgotten to take my EpiPen anywhere with me.

As few as twenty-five years ago, only at the absurdist theatre would one expect to meet such a family—a family which lives in constant fear of a small, crunchy hunk of cellulose. Unfortunately, this has become strange reality for many more families than my own.

"Anaphylactic" literally means defenseless; giants though we are, the smallest particle has the power to topple us. For an anaphylactic, the shadow of death skulks in the silliest places: vending machines, refrigerators, ice-cream parlors, and parks where nice old ladies feed squirrels. The mundane randomness of the peanut, as well as milk, eggs, and other embarrassingly benign foods that our bodies lethally reject, allow them to slip beneath the radar of the common mind. People appear to have an easier time empathizing with a diabetic or cancer patient—diseases where the enemy is one's own body, which must be constantly moderated, used gingerly, and plied with medicine; a situation we've all experienced in times of illness. However, to the average onlooker I imagine an anaphylactic must look like a barefoot Achilles carefully avoiding sharp stones on the ground, or King Stefan of *Sleeping Beauty* obsessively purging his kingdom of doomful spinning wheels. Oftentimes, I feel embarrassed about how silly my own requests for accommodation sound. After a new acquaintance has invited me into his home for the first time, I find myself asking him to move a bag of mixed nuts from the living room to the kitchen. If he doesn't answer my request, instead of insisting I just move to the far end of the couch, and take care not to touch my face with my fingers for the rest of the night.

My best anaphylaxis story (I say that only half-ironically) is about the first time I had dinner at my girlfriend's house. Like the careful person she was, she instructed her parents not to cook with any nuts. Needless to say, it is rather uncouth to kill your daughter's boyfriend. We sat down and I began to endure the sincere rituals of meeting the parents. I then noticed that I had begun to have an allergic reaction—how awkward. Since my girlfriend had assured me that no nut products (and especially, no peanuts) had entered the meal, I suspected that it was likely just an accidental sliver of almond that had snuck into the lamb or the salad, and I resolved to silently weather my reaction for the sake of my relationship with her parents. They were native Chinese; China being a country where allergy rates have historically been miniscule. I didn't want to cause a fuss over an itchy throat, so I would just eat around . . . whatever it was that I had eaten. Almost half an hour later, after the meal (with dessert, no less!), I felt nauseous, so I excused myself to the upstairs bathroom. Looking in the mirror, I observed that I was bright red. I was up against no mere almond.

Five minutes later, her father was racing me to the hospital. I did my best to keep her calm as we sat in the back seat, even as my face gradually became more inflated and hideous in front of her.

The instigating food item had been a precooked onion pancake that been cooked in peanut oil. I had eaten the same dish, cooked in different oil, a week earlier, and presumed this time it would also be safe. It was an honest mistake on their part; perhaps they had never experienced eating with an allergic person before.

I survived the event, as any adequately prepared anaphylactic would (thanks for reminding me to bring my EpiPen, mum). I was able to keep cool the entire time because I had done it before (I hadn't died any of the other times), and I figured my luck would hold out this time as well. And hold out it did—my girlfriend later told me I had impressed her father with my stoicism.

That incident was the fourth time I had almost been killed by my condition. (There has since been a fifth, which my mother won't know about until she reads this preface I've written here.) I've already accepted it as something that would happen to me from time to time, like a monkey learning that tigers are a fact of the forest. I've been content my entire life constrained in my circumstances simply because I've known nothing else.

Besides, there are plenty who have it much worse than me. There are cases of children who must be carefully isolated, usually entailing homeschooling, because they are sensitive to such a vast array of things (they will likely live in a bubble for their entire lives). At least I have the luxury of being able to visit my girlfriend's parents' house—and the luxury of being unafraid to touch door-knobs.

Whereas I've always been very nonchalant in my approach to my allergy, my mother has refused to accept my absurd reality at every turn. For many years, she's been battling the notion that this is the way that things must be.

Young people, myself included, tend to think of ourselves as unkillable pro-tagonists covered in impenetrable plot armor. Parents are smarter than their children; they have been the narrators that kept their main characters from dying throughout their childhood and they have known just how easy it can be to lose something. Any risk factors must be eliminated; that's why my mom cares so much about getting to the root of this phenomenon. Even if it's too late for her to live a motherhood without the constant threat of losing a child, and too late for me to live a childhood where I get to eat peanuts (I expect they taste amazing, or you all would have no excuse for eating them), perhaps we can help the parents of the future and make a world without bubble children or Sabrina Shannons.

Since 1990, the peanut-allergic population of the United States has more than tripled, now numbering a tragic three million individuals. We know how to treat it, we know how to mitigate it, but we still haven't agreed on what causes it, let alone figured out how to cure it. Large-scale anaphylaxis has not always been a fact. Anaphylaxis occurs rarely in many parts of the world; this may indicate a short-term, likely human cause historically unique to westernized countries. If this is the case, it is baffling that we haven't discovered it already.

Woodrow Fraser-Boychuk holds a BA in creative writing & English language and literature from Western University.

Introduction

THE PROBLEM OF
PEANUT ALLERGY

By 2012, as many as 2.3% of Canadian children under 18 and 2% to 3% of children in the US, the UK and AU were allergic to peanut. (See Appendix). And as children born during the first wave of the epidemic in the early 1990s have aged, the statistic of adults with peanut allergy is increasing. In 2008, an estimated 1% of the US population was allergic to this one food, about 3 million people. Four years later by 2012, that number jumped to an estimated 4 million living with a life threatening allergy to peanuts.

Peanut allergy began as a phenomenon largely affecting children living in Western countries, the US, Canada, Australia and the UK. The alarm sounded for Americans when between 1997 and 2002 the number of peanut allergic children doubled and then tripled reaching an astonishing one million in 2008. In 2010 one study put that number at 2%, an additional 500,000 children in just two years. As this book unfolds it will become evident that there is a pattern in the way in which the peanut allergy in Western and now non-Western countries has emerged—epidemic levels of peanut allergy in children are now also documented in mainland China, Hong Kong, Singapore, Israel and parts of Africa.

While the exact numbers are a matter of debate, it is clear through statistics, scientific inquiry, and simple anecdotal evidence (the parental refrain "no one had a peanut allergy when I was at school") that the prevalence of the allergy among children has increased at an *alarming* rate.[1] This development has altered the fabric of societies now forced to accommodate life-threatening allergies to common foods.

Families with children allergic to peanuts (or any of the other top 8 allergenic foods—tree nuts, fish, shellfish, wheat, soy, dairy, egg)[2] live in a state of constant tension. If these families eat at restaurants, they do so with extreme caution. Not knowing the severity of the allergy, parents are vigilant about smears of peanut butter left on tables or on grocery cart handles. Trace amounts on the skin or lip or even the scent of the food could trigger a reaction. Parents, the child, caregivers, and teachers are fearful. Children are segregated in school cafeterias at designated tables or left out of play because friends have peanut butter in the house. Every school now tackles the peanut question, whether to ban peanut butter sandwiches and how to educate staff and students about the deadly nature of this ubiquitous childhood food.

Public awareness of peanut and other severe food allergies has impacted education systems and social norms, provoked legal reform, and made billions of dollars for those active in the food-allergy industry. This industry's infrastructure consists of many overlapping allergy awareness groups, international allergy associations, medical researchers, pharmaceutical companies, allergy doctors, "free from" food makers, and government regulators, all of which support or are supported by the growing legions of food-allergic children.

The inherent inertia of this industrious leviathan, however, has pushed the salient questions into the background: How has the peanut allergy epidemic developed, and why is it continuing?

It is difficult to accept the startling increase in peanut allergies in children in just the last twenty years as a coincidence or to chalk it up to genetic fluke. The challenge for any concerned medical professional has been to unearth the precise practical mechanism of sensitization common to these children—how did they become sensitized to peanut in the first place? And while there are a limited number of proven ways of "how to" make someone anaphylactic—ingestion, inhalation, through the skin, injection—no hypothesis of *mass sensitization* has yet connected any of these functional mechanisms to all the specific characteristics of the peanut-allergy epidemic.

Researchers have considered skin creams that contain peanut oil, peanut consumption, parasite burden, and more without satisfactorily explaining why there has been a rise of the allergy in children. Why peanut? Why has it happened so suddenly, and why just in certain countries, most of them Western?

Risk factors for developing the allergy have been explored without conclusion. These include the following: maternal age, mode of delivery, levels of intestinal flora, heredity, and even birth month and socioeconomic status. Confusing matters further is a debate over the basic concept of allergy: Is allergy the outcome of a roulette-style genetic predisposition to immune dysfunction, or is allergy an innate, purposeful immune defense?

An important and clear distinction must be made between *sensitizing* someone to peanut and *launching* the allergic reaction. Sensitization is believed to occur when a protein bypasses the detoxifying process of the digestive system and becomes bonded with blood serum. This prompts specific blood cells to create antibodies that are then programmed to recognize the threatening protein—in this case, peanut protein. The launching of an allergic reaction, on the other hand, occurs when the body is subsequently exposed to the protein and the antibodies trigger the biochemical players in the allergic reaction.

Lack of a standardized definition of anaphylaxis has hampered some studies where categories of "true" anaphylaxis mediated by Ig antibodies are compared with non-Ig anaphylaxis. This is less of a concern with peanut allergy where apparent consensus is that it is almost always Ig mediated.

Immunoglobulins epsilon (called IgE) are sentries of the body. The job of the IgE is to patrol the fortress walls—mucous membranes—looking for peanut protein intruders. When they detect one of the many peanut protein epitopes (strings of amino acids that are numbered 1 through 8 and all called Ara h after *Arachis hypogea*, Latin for peanut)[3] they alert the body, which in turn lets loose the army—the body's immune system. A biochemical cascade is deployed that is damaging and potentially dangerous. It is typically characterized by coughing, shortness of breath, itchy skin hives, systemic leaking of blood vessels that causes swelling and potential asphyxia, vomiting, and diarrhea. In severe reactions, blood pressure drops, draining vital organs and causing the heart to stop.

Scientists have shown that the anaphylactic condition in all mammals can be achieved by inhaling peanut protein if it is combined with a toxic additive. For example, doctors have created anaphylaxis in lab animals that inhaled a mixture of peanut and cholera.[4] The toxic bacteria functions as an adjuvant, an additive that excites the immune system to form antibodies. It is suggested that the toxin and benign food can become in this way linked and both remembered by the immune system.[5] One wonders then at the idea of an allergy to bacteria and the toxins produced by them. Allergy to bacterial toxins has been acknowledged for many years[6] and can result in inflammation of the tonsils and adenoids[7] and anaphylaxis.[8]

Researchers have not explored the role of adjuvants in peanut sensitization. They have preferred to focus only on the peanut proteins, their allergenicity, and the ingestion of them as the most obvious elements in sensitization. They seemed to think that if they could simply pinpoint the initial oral exposure to these proteins, they could stop the epidemic. To this end, they have considered the ways in which peanuts are prepared (boiled versus roasted), age when they are introduced to the child's diet, maternal diet and breast milk, and even peanut oil used in nipple creams. Although it is possible to create the condition through simple ingestion, it is difficult. A healthy digestive system will neutralize any potentially sensitizing protein.

In fact, a 2006–2007 study stated that it did not matter whether mothers ate peanuts or not—the same percentage of children developed the allergy. Some children whose mothers did not eat peanuts before, during, or after pregnancy still developed a peanut allergy. Kids who had never been exposed to peanuts exhibited anaphylaxis on their first or second taste of it—suggesting that they were already sensitized either to peanut proteins or to proteins similar enough to them leading to cross-reactivity. Adding to the allergy mystery is the fact that Sweden, which has a low level of peanut consumption, has a higher prevalence of the allergy than the United States. Israel, which has a high level of peanut consumption, has a low prevalence of peanut allergy in Jewish children at .6% in 2012 (but a high prevalence of sesame allergy) and a high prevalence of peanut allergy in Arab children (2.6%) living in the same country.

Another puzzling feature of the epidemic is the sudden emergence of peanut allergy in non-Westernized countries like Ghana, China and Singapore. It was suggested previously by Sampson et al in 2001 that children living in China did not have peanut allergy because their peanuts are boiled which partially destroys and reduces sensitizing peanut proteins. However, the sudden and increasing prevalence of food allergy in children living in mainland China and peanut allergy Hong Kong upends this theory and deepens the seeming mystery of this allergy.

Today, thousands of research articles by doctors on the biology of the allergic reaction, clinical observations, and allergy management are available in prestigious periodicals. From this mound of information, doctors have developed and tend to favor two explanations for the current epidemic of peanut-sensitized children. They are the helminth hypothesis and the hygiene hypothesis.

Helminths are worms that live in the human intestinal tract. It surprised researchers in the 1980s to discover that people heavily infected with worms had few allergies. One study confirmed that most Venezuelan Indians living in the rainforest had worms but no allergies while very few of the wealthy Venezuelans living in the cities had worm infections, but many had allergies.

From this observation, researchers developed an explanation for all allergies: because parasites and humans have coevolved, they have an apparent symbiotic relationship in which parasites suppress allergic reactions while enjoying their human host. Without worms, the theory states, humans are unable to achieve homeostasis. In other words, immune dysfunction occurs due to lack of worms.

As an explanation for peanut allergy, the helminth hypothesis is inadequate. It cannot explain why there has been a rise of peanut allergy just in children. And given that Western countries have been largely unburdened by major helminth infections for decades, it does not explain the sudden increase of food allergy that shocked school systems in the early 1990s.

Another popular explanation for the rise in childhood allergies grew from an apparent correlation between this rise and the general decline in family size. It was proposed that unhygienic contact in large families—lots of siblings bringing illness home from school—was important for the development of a healthy immune system. The greatly expanded and much-touted hygiene hypothesis suggests that overzealous cleaning, germ-killing products, chlorinated water, antibiotics, (vaccination is specifically avoided by researchers) have "protected" Western children unnaturally. And as a result, the immune systems of First World children, in particular, are sheltered from a natural microbial burden. Their immature immune systems are understimulated, dysregulated, and therefore prone to random allergic sensitization. This malfunction is a product of an unburdened lifestyle.

The hygiene hypothesis is problematic in explaining peanut allergy. It does not consider the possibility that the immune systems of these children are not understimulated but rather overstimulated by Westernized approaches to toxic chemicals, drugs, and vaccinations. In addition, the theory does not indicate a practical mechanism of mass sensitization that would explain the sharp rise in food allergy just in children that was first noticed in the early 1990s in specific countries when a flood of affected children arrived for kindergarten.

This is a primary clue to causation that researchers have either missed or dismissed altogether.

In addition, these two favored explanations for the epidemic assume that allergy is a dysfunction, that the body has made a mistake in attacking a benign substance. And yet, the opposite may be true. Some suggest that allergy has an evolved purpose seen before the twentieth century but provoked increasingly today by drugs and noxious pollutants in our air, water, and food.

American researchers Rachel Carson (1907–1964) and Theron G. Randolph (1906–1995) and evolutionary biologist Margie Profet (b. 1958) proposed that allergy is an evolved protective response. In 1991, Profet stated in *The Function of Allergy* that allergy is a final and often risky natural defense against toxins linked to benign substances. The IgE antibody is not, as it is generally characterized in medical literature, a rogue immune factor.[9] It is more akin to a hero provoked by toxins the body has deemed a deadly threat. The scratching, vomiting, diarrhea, and sneezing are desperate attempts to eject a toxin as fast as possible. It is a risky reaction but one the body is programmed to unleash as a last-ditch effort to protect itself. This event occurs when the general defenses have been insufficient in preventing a specific toxin from accessing the bloodstream for a second time.

This is a provocative concept. However, because it was developed before the rise in peanut allergy, it lacks specificity—again, why peanut and why the sudden increased prevalence in children?

Conspicuous by its absence from current theories is the one mechanism that has an actual history of creating mass allergy—injection. Injection is examined in this book in some detail since it was the means by which the founder of anaphylaxis, Dr. Charles Richet, stumbled on alimentary (food) anaphylaxis in humans and animals over one hundred years ago. Richet concluded in 1913 that food anaphylaxis was a response to proteins that had evaded modification by the digestive system. Using a hypodermic needle, he was able to create the condition in a variety of animals—mammals and amphibians—proving that the reaction was not only universal but also predictable using the method of injection followed by consumption or another injection.

There are two lines of thought in the medical literature regarding injection as a mechanism of sensitization. The first is that injection, in the form of vaccination or other injections such as the neonatal vitamin K1 prophylaxis, merely *unmasks* genetic predispositions or tendencies to allergic disease. In short, there is something wrong with the child and not the injection(s).

The second line of thought is that there is a causal relationship between the injected ingredients and allergy—and although the proven allergenicity of vaccines is widely acknowledged, medical literature carefully avoids the question of what kinds of allergies vaccines can and do create to substances that are coincidentally or subsequently inhaled, ingested or injected. One exception to this unwritten rule was an unusual admission by Japanese doctors that an outbreak of gelatin allergy in children starting in 1988 and continuing through the 1990s was caused by pediatric vaccination. In that year, changes to the vaccination schedule in Japan meant that the DTP was replaced by an acellular version containing gelatin, the age at which it was administered to children was dropped from two years to three months, and this new vaccine was given before the live virus MMR vaccine that also contained gelatin. When children began reacting with anaphylaxis to the MMR vaccine as well as gelatin-containing foods (yogurt, Jell-O, etc.), doctors investigated. Finally, they concluded that the aluminum adjuvant in the DTaP had helped sensitize children to the "minute amounts" of proteins in the refined gelatin in the vaccine. Removal of gelatin from the DTaP vaccines was "an ultimate solution for vaccine-related gelatin allergy."[10] Subsequently, new cases of gelatin allergy in Japanese children dropped.

Quantities and qualities of adjuvant and other vaccine ingredients injected into children changed dramatically between 1989 and 1994 in 'mature markets' for vaccines including the United States, United Kingdom, Canada, and Australia. During those years, at least five new vaccine formulations for the same bacteria, *Haemophilus influenzae* type b (Hib) were introduced within an expanded and intense vaccination schedule. Like the gelatin allergy that emerged from a changed schedule of pediatric injections, was there some mix of ingredients that included powerful aluminum additives in the new Western schedule that was sensitizing children to peanut? The fact that refined peanut oil was a documented vaccine ingredient in the past is a subject of concern equal to the potential of sensitization to body tissues or even of cross-reactivity between dietary peanut and homologous injected proteins. These cross-reactive proteins may include those in the Hib cellular membrane or legume oil in a popular brand of the vitamin K1 prophylaxis. Cross-reactivity explains why a person who is allergic to peanuts, legumes like soy and castor beans, may also react to nuts or citrus seeds,[11] which belong to different plant families—their proteins have similar molecular weights and structures.

As ingredients changed, the number of shots increased for kids in their first eighteen months of life from ten to as many as twenty-nine. The increase meant inconvenience to parents who would have to make more trips to the doctor and discomfort to the children who would have to experience multiple injections. To overcome these obstacles to compliance with the new schedule, the vaccines for diphtheria, pertussis, and tetanus (DPT); polio (OPV); and *H. influenzae* b (Hib) were administered to children in a single visit with two injections and an oral polio dose starting around 1988. By 1994 starting in Canada, these five were rolled into a single needle. Few parents realize that by design, immunization provokes both the desired immune response and allergy at the same time. These natural defenses are inseparable and the more potent the vaccine, the more powerful the two responses. This is an outcome of vaccination the medical community has understood at least since Charles Richet won the Nobel Prize (1913) for his research on anaphylaxis. Anaphylaxis, Richet observed, is one of three outcomes of vaccination.

Paul Offit, chief of Infectious Diseases at Children's Hospital in Philadelphia in 2008, dismissed concerns that the vaccination schedule was overwhelming children. To Offit, this was just not good science.[12] Other doctors disagreed. In respected medical journals such as *The Journal of the American Medical Association* and *Allergy: European Journal of Allergy and Clinical Immunology*, doctors expressed concern over the long-term effects of early vaccinations.[13] Some doctors state that excessive vaccination is ineffective and dangerous.[14]

But vaccination is a complex subject, and its role in the food-allergy epidemic is difficult to address because of the heated political, social, and economic implications. It is a subject doctors avoid. And so, despite the continuing intense attention given to the peanut allergy in children, an answer to its cause(s) has not yet been found. What has emerged, instead, is a robust economy of doctor fees, nut-free foods, ongoing medical research, and pharmaceutical sales. Peanut and other food allergies have become enormously profitable. It is so much so that one market analyst has suggested that an "autoimmune index" would be a great tool for investors. This index, tagged as "save the children and make money," would monitor the profitability of pharmaceutical stocks relative to the continued rise in peanut allergy and other childhood epidemics.[15]

Peanut allergy began as a mere idiosyncrasy after World War II. Today, its epidemic proportions help fuel a multibillion-dollar food-allergy industry.

Part 1

THE MYSTERY OF THE PEANUT ALLERGY EPIDEMIC

Chapter 1

—⚬⚬⚬—

FROM IDIOSYNCRASY TO MULTIBILLION-DOLLAR INDUSTRY

Thirty-year-old Dr. Walter Teller disembarked from the Holland American liner *Maasdam* at New York City in December 1954. Traveling from Germany, the young doctor had accepted a position at Mercy Hospital in Altoona, Pennsylvania, and was greeted by his new colleagues at the pier. The men went to dinner in midtown. Five hours later, Dr. Teller was "nearly strangled" when his esophagus closed. He had eaten peanuts for the first time.

While a contemporary account of this event—possibly the first peanut reaction to be reported in the popular media—would reflect drama, fear, and worry that a doctor could be so blithe about peanuts, at the time it was barely newsworthy. To the reporter who covered the story in five paragraphs, the allergic reaction was about as interesting as the doctor's car that, coincidentally, had been vandalized during that very dinner. Dr. Teller's unusual first evening in New York City was buried on page 31 in the Books section of *The New York Times*.[1]

Until the last decade of the twentieth century, the US press typically met the rare and curious reactions to peanut with surprise and a shrug of the shoulders. It was just too hard to imagine that a common food could really be that dangerous even to the obvious victim. A rare feature on allergy in *Harper's Magazine* in

1939 delved into the defensive nature of these strange "food idiosyncrasies" that could cause swelling, sneezing, headaches, itching, and rash, but not death it seemed.[2] In fact, allergy had a lighter side. A young woman's allergy helped her prove that a platinum necklace from her fickle sweetheart was actually nickel when she broke out in an allergic rash. And a restaurant patron proved by virtue of his swollen ankles that the economic waiter had merely scraped the anchovies off his eggs before re-serving them.

At this time, however, there was one exception to the anomalous nature of food allergies. Starting in the late 1930s, there was a small but troubling outbreak of anaphylaxis to just one food—cottonseed oil. The outbreak startled doctors, government agencies, and the food industry but, again, was not newsworthy. In the few reports about allergy at this time, cottonseed oil was mentioned as just one among many foods that could cause reactions.[3]

In an investigation, however, the Food and Drug Administration (FDA) found that sloppy cottonseed-crushing protocols had led to the contamination of many other oils subsequently used in processed foods. While this discovery explained how people were exposed unknowingly to the oil, it did not explain how so many had suddenly become sensitized to it. They had been consuming this oil for decades in the United States without apparent problem. Doctors responded to the outbreak with a flurry of analyses and opinions none of which managed to unearth the functional cause of this mass sensitization.[4]

The rising prevalence of cottonseed allergy, however, resolved as quickly and as mysteriously as it had arrived.[5] Intense scrutiny in medical literature of this outbreak peaked during the late 1940s and sharply declined during the 1950s. This short-lived medical crisis was never fully investigated.

As reports of cottonseed allergy fell, peanut allergy emerged in US medical literature. Prevalence of this allergy, however, grew more slowly.

In 1941, well-known allergist Warren Vaughan, in his book *Strange Malady*, had dismissed peanut from his considerable list of potential food allergens. In his medical practice, Vaughan had seen allergies to milk, egg, corn, soybean, cottonseed, shrimp, tomato, cabbage, cherry, chocolate, strawberries, and many more foods. Significantly, however, the doctor did not consider there to be any allergic concern about peanut. In fact, in the book he mentioned crushed peanuts as a food topping without further comment. And yet, by 1948, peanut sensitivity had become a serious obstacle in studies involving children and penicillin that contained a peanut oil additive.[6]

Medical articles published in 1956, 1961, and 1963 reveal a growing interest in the increasingly common allergy to peanuts.[7] Peanut and other severe food allergies soon affected so many people that with the peanut allergy death in 1972 of a ten-year-old Boston boy, Michael Grzybinski, there was a public outcry for proper food-container labeling.

The media coverage of this tragedy revealed a far greater sympathy for food-allergic people than had been exhibited in the 1950s over Dr. Teller's near-death experience. The death of a child who had eaten "ice cream with peanut butter whipped into it" might have been prevented if the container had had its ingredients listed on the side, exclaimed a very upset Dr. Jean Mayer, professor of nutrition at Harvard University. The doctor wrote the following: "We think food manufacturers should no more be allowed to hide behind 'the need to protect recipe secrets' than drug manufacturers are. In both cases, lack of information can be not only unhealthy, but even deadly."[8]

The doctor's anger in albeit the limited press coverage is matched only by the sadness of the parents who, in an open letter, demanded that the FDA implement labeling laws. A deepening awareness of peanut as a deadly problem for a slim minority of children and adults found more room in newspapers from that moment on. Yet, the allergy was still not taken seriously. Throughout the 1970s, peanut allergy in the media was isolated to festive occasions like Christmas. Newspaper food section articles alerted the conscientious hostess to the potential of food allergy among her holiday guests. Peanut allergy was not a cause for widespread alarm.

And yet, doctors knew it was on the rise.

In 1973, the first formal US study of peanut allergy was launched by S. A. Bock who followed 114 children for twelve years, concluding that none had outgrown his or her reactivity.[9] The report underlined the fact that children were developing food anaphylaxis at an unusual rate and that peanut had emerged as a dangerous food that should be watched.[10] And so doctors watched the allergy, none publicly posing the obvious question—like the cottonseed oil mystery, what was causing people to become sensitized to this one food? An additional and surprising question this time, however, was why the allergy appeared to have an increased impact on children.

But rather than unearth the root cause of this mounting concern, doctors in 1980 chose instead to address the allergy after it had been established. In that year, medical researchers isolated the proteins that trigger the peanut reaction—Ara h

1 and 2. This was valuable information in the manufacturing of vaccines and other allergy treatments. The growing problem of peanut and other food allergies was a market opportunity for pharmaceutical companies.

In 1980, the EpiPen was introduced to allergists who prescribed them for patients. The EpiPen is a portable emergency autoinjection of epinephrine. Epinephrine temporarily relaxes muscles and slows the allergic reaction. The EpiPen automatic syringe was licensed to Center Laboratories, New York, from manufacturer Survival Technology Inc. (STI) owned by physician Stanley J. Sarnoff. STI and inventor Shel Kaplan had patented the hypodermic injection device in 1977. The syringe was originally designed for the US military to supplement STI's other autoinjector that was used to administer a nerve gas antidote during battle.[11]

Commercial interests led the way in allergy management while social, legal, and political initiatives lagged. Poor food labeling, again, was blamed for another death in 1980 of a seventeen-year-old boy. He had eaten a candy bar that contained peanuts.[12]

A turning point in media sympathy for peanut-allergic children was marked by the death of an eighteen-year-old US national squash champion in 1986.[13] This tragedy was followed by a new tone of sober inquiry into what the media perceived to be a serious and growing threat to children. A healthy and accomplished teenager had died after eating a spoonful of chili thickened with peanut butter. Headlines reflected new vigor in bringing information to the public, including population studies and a review of emergency measures.

The media challenged restaurants to list ingredients and airlines to consider in-flight peanut restrictions.[14] Of new import for the first time was interest in an explanation for this child-specific allergy—thoughts turned naturally to mothers' diets while pregnant and breastfeeding. In 1941, allergist Warren Vaughan had already fingered the "abnormal food cravings"[15] of pregnant women as the source of allergens to which children often become sensitized. But this educated guesswork did not explain the rising prevalence of allergy to peanuts when this dietary staple had been consumed for decades without obvious problem—in fact, again, Vaughan had outright dismissed peanut from his list of food allergens. By 1987, however, one reporter looked fearfully to an allergy-filled future following the death of an eleven-year-old asthmatic boy who had eaten peanut-contaminated cake: "Every week brings reports of new dangers, a death from allergy."[16]

Refreshed marketing efforts for EpiPens in 1988 introduced the word *anaphylaxis* to the mainstream media. News reports for the lifesaving emergency device exploited the story of the 1986 death from peanut butter–"laced" chili. An EpiPen might have saved the teen's life. An article to this effect ran in the newspapers of six US cities in the summer of 1988.[17]

Starting around 1990, the media buzzed about EpiPens, new allergy guides, cookbooks, labeling concerns, holiday season dangers, and the biology of "when your immune system panics."[18] People began to question if the allergy could be passed via organ transplant, and even whether the allergy was an overdiagnosed malady,[19] when the prevalence of peanut allergy in children suddenly accelerated. Unnoticed by the public, hospital emergency room (ER) records in Australia, the United Kingdom, and the United States documented the upward momentum of food anaphylaxis admissions for children under five.

In the United States, ER records showed a steady and rapid increase in anaphylaxis discharges between 1992 and 1994 from 467 per 100,000 to 671. This number jumped to 876 in 1995. In three years from 1992–95 the numbers nearly doubled. A 1991 US study determined that 90% of all food allergy fatalities were due to ingestion of peanut/tree nuts.[20]

In the Australian Capital Territory (ACT), a fourfold increase in hospital admission rates for food allergy was observed from 1993 through 2004–5. ACT is a self-governing state within New South Wales with the highest density population and smallest area at 910 square miles. Within it is the national capital of Canberra. A twelve-year study of allergy services in ACT showed a 400% increase for this period for children under five. During the course of the study, birth rates actually fell 10%. One allergist in Australia referred to this trend in allergy in children as an epidemic.[21]

In hindsight, what was called the tip of the iceberg[22] by University of Edinburgh allergist Aziz Sheikh in a 2006 lecture, the discharge rates for system allergic disorder in England increased between 1990 and 2001 from 1,960 admissions for allergic conditions to 6,752. This threefold jump in just eleven years indicated "a highly significant increase" in admissions for severe allergy.

The timing of this acceleration was confirmed by a UK peanut allergy study. A retrospective cohort analysis of children born between January 1989 and February 1990 on the Isle of Wight revealed a shocking statistic: by ages four and five in 1994, 0.5% of these children were anaphylactic to peanut and 1.1% showed sensitivity to it.[23]

This news made riveting headlines. Not only were 40,000 UK children under four years of age "in peril from peanuts," but they could also react as one child did, to just its vapor.[24] A 1997 issue of London's *Sunday Times Magazine* sensationalized the sudden new threat to children in "One Bite and He Dies."[25]

A second cohort analysis from the Isle of Wight provided an even bigger shock. An analysis of children born in the same region between September 1, 1994, and August 31, 1996, and tested at ages three and four, revealed that twice as many children were now allergic to peanuts: 1.1% were anaphylactic, and 3.3% were sensitized.[26] Newspapers again heralded the "rise of the killer food."[27] Allergies to peanuts in UK preschoolers had more than doubled in just four years, and no one knew why.

Two other startling facts emerged around this time. The first was that 6% of Americans had "serologic evidence" of sensitivity to peanuts according to the US Centers for Disease Control's (CDC) National Health and Nutrition Examination Survey (NHANE III data was collected from 1988 to 1994).[28] In other words, about fourteen million people in the United States had somehow become sensitized to peanut even if they were not actively reacting.

The second fact was that peanut allergy at this time appeared to be a concern only in Western countries. In China, for example, where peanut consumption was as high as in the West, the allergy was virtually unknown. Researchers suggested that the difference lay in the way peanuts were prepared. The Chinese often boiled their peanuts[29] that reduced their allergenicity while Americans roasted their peanuts, a process that intensified it. This explanation had many problems not least of which was that if both countries had been eating peanuts for decades without seeming problem, why the sudden prevalence in reactivity, and why were children increasingly at risk for the allergy? As well, the mode of preparation theory did not hold true for India where peanut was prepared in a variety of ways, including roasting, and where the allergy was also not known at this time to exist.

While the mystery deepened, doctors continued to focus on postsensitization treatments such as vaccination and allergy shots. Both treatments were fraught with problems given the potential severity of the allergy.[30] A 1991 desensitizing experiment in Denver was nearly derailed by an accidental death. While it was reported that three patients in the study experienced diminished reactions to peanut after their shots, a fifteen-year-old boy died when he received an incorrect injection dosage.[31] A pharmacist received two years probation for this death.

Looking back from 2006, allergist Hugh Sampson was quoted as saying that in this and other such trials, "everybody was getting significant adverse reactions throughout. So it was decided that standard immunotherapy was not a reasonable way to go."[32]

The "ultimate allergy shot" was made public in January 1995 by Peptide Therapeutics in the United Kingdom.[33] It was potentially "one of the biggest selling drugs ever." The company had already raised £4.5 million and was ready for human clinical trials. A news report explained that the vaccine worked by provoking the body to generate IgG antibodies that suppress IgE, the allergy antibodies. The UK vaccine, however, appeared to fall from the spotlight as quickly as it had emerged.

Later in the United States, research and clinical trials using a vaccine TNX-901 to reduce sensitivity to peanut were ultimately axed during a much-publicized squabble over rights between two pharmaceutical giants.[34]

Meanwhile, EpiPen sales were growing. In 1992, Center Labs in New York paired with Fisons Pharmaceuticals to distribute marketing material that claimed 15% of the US population—38 million people—who had life-threatening allergies to drugs and foods.[35] They were all reached by their team of 350 sales reps visiting primary care physicians and pediatricians across the United States. Their smaller sales team of fifteen would continue to sell to allergy doctors. EpiPen ads appeared in medical journals like the *Journal of the American Medical Association* (*JAMA*). Retailing at $30 in 1992, about four hundred thousand EpiPens were sold in the United States, and the marketers hoped to sell one million more over the next two years for gross sales of $15 million.[36] The North American retail price of an EpiPen was between $64 and $118 in 2009. By 2014, the retail price was upwards of $330. for two, sold as a package. Gross annual sales of EpiPens in 2012 was $640 million.

A real comprehension of the danger posed by peanut to a minority of children dawned more slowly on public school staff members. In 1994, a frightened mother learned that a lunchroom aide at her son's elementary school had forced her six-year-old peanut-allergic son to bite a nut cookie.[37] The private UN International School in New York made headlines when a peanut-allergic five-year-old was denied entry after his mother refused to sign a waiver of responsibility.[38] One creative allergist and a mom of an allergic two-year-old thought allergy badges might help at schools and day cares. Shirts emblazoned with badges of bright yellow, green, and pink would single out the fatally allergic.[39] This double-edged idea did not catch on. Doctors had warned of psychological issues related to wearing EpiPen belts and badges would be no less problematic.

Peanut allergy tipped into critical mass in the early 1990s when a "sudden surge of severely allergic children entering school systems . . . caught many educators off guard."[40] A 2000 article published in a magazine for Canadian teachers recounted the surprising phenomenon of the unexpected flood of four- and five-year-old food-allergic children. In that same year, the principal of an elementary school in the Hastings and Prince Edward District School Board, Ontario, was aware of the rising number of anaphylactic children she saw in the schools. On her own initiative, she conducted an ad hoc survey of elementary schools in her board to confirm the numbers. It was a quiet survey intended as a communication between principals only, but it made its way to a local anaphylaxis support group. The principal's findings were shocking. The document titled "Severe Life-Threatening Allergies, Survey Results" (September 2000) revealed that in twenty-six responding schools there were eighty-six children with anaphylaxis. In these twenty-six schools, forty children born between 1987 and 1996 were allergic to nuts and another thirty were allergic to bee stings. This report remained buried in a filing cabinet until 2011.

Schools were obliged by law to deal with the enormous social, medical, and logistical problems of protecting handfuls of peanut- and other food-allergic kindergarten children in each school. There were thousands of these children across school boards, and soon there were hundreds of thousands across the United States, Canada, and other Westernized countries. This eyewitness to the surge confirmed by ER records plus the Isle of Wight cohort studies pointed to these few years—the late 1980s and early '90s—as the starting point of the accelerated prevalence of peanut allergy in children. Society was unaware that anything had happened until the affected children showed up for kindergarten.

By 1996, some schools had created peanut-free zones while others attempted to ban peanuts altogether as they did in Massachusetts.[41] One school in North Andover that banned peanuts had five kindergarten students with peanut allergy. These kids were assigned to the same peanut-free class, all substances—including the hand soap—were checked for hidden ingredients, and all parents were told to leave the peanut butter at home. And yet, some felt the peanut ban was not the best solution. "Peanut bans don't work," stated Ann Munoz-Furlong in 1996, founder of the Food Allergy and Anaphylaxis Network (FAAN).[42] A peanut-free status suggested to people that they were safe "and that's dangerous. They let their guard down."

Most schools, however, did not have policies or procedures, and certainly there were no laws. In this unprotected vacuum, parents grew fearful and refused to let their allergic kids attend field trips, envisioning their reactive child trapped on a bus with the food. These parents strapped Epi-belts on the children and taught them how to use the autoinjector, not yet trusting schools to have this medication at the ready. They profiled their allergic children in laminated homemade posters placed strategically in schools.

Most kindergarten children ate their lunches in their classroom, so initially, only individual classrooms were made peanut-free. As more allergic children entered school behind the initial group, they were accommodated in lunchrooms with separate tables.

Lunch-bag inspections became common. Any peanut-related food, granola bar, or sandwich was confiscated and sent home with a cautionary note. At some of Toronto's peanut-free schools in 2009, any child with a food item that "may contain" peanut or nut was segregated at the Peanut Table. Peanut allergy had become the new normal, and peanut products a politically incorrect choice at Ontario schools.

But ten years earlier in the late 1990s, parents of peanut-allergic children incurred the enmity of the, as yet, not-understanding parents of the nonallergic children. This latter group of parents insisted that the peanut butter ban had violated their rights. "A staple was under fire," screamed a 1996 headline.[43] Peanut butter, a cheap and tasty source of protein, had been a staple of lunch boxes for decades. Eventually, more and more schools went peanut free with varying degrees of success given the enormity of the task.

In 1998, concern related to children with peanut and nut allergies noticeably impacted family grocery-buying habits—the growth of the "free from" food market category was a concrete index of the epidemic having hit critical mass. That year, the Swiss-based food giant Nestlé responded to this market reality with a line of chocolate bars made in a "peanut-free facility." Targeting concerned adults, Nestlé marketed their "peanut-free promise" with Halloween food safety.

Halloween generates the greatest sales volume of sweets for the entire year. According to a Nielsen market report, chocolate sales in 2008 accounted for $1.2

billion of the total $1.9 billion of candy sales. In 2001, forty-one million trick-or-treaters filled their bags with candy. Other savvy food manufacturers soon jumped on board with allergen-free products for children (cookies, candy, ice cream) and cautious labeling.

The peanut segment of the snack market fell from 14.4% to 12.4% between 1993 and 1999. The shrinking supply-managed peanut industry[44] remained sluggish in large part due to the growth in peanut-allergy concerns.[45] The important youth market segment of children under fourteen was in decline. In 2008, it was recommended that peanut industry leaders not wait for the health care industry to fix the allergy problem and to take matters into their own hands by producing a transgenic, allergen-free peanut.

In 2003, biotech giant Monsanto began to grow genetically engineered peanuts in India. By 2007,[46] these peanuts were approved for growth in the United States by the American Peanut Council. Urging due diligence on the part of scientists, the council claimed that an engineered peanut could be safer, more nutritious, and easier to grow than conventional versions. At Georgia University, Peggy Ozias-Akins, a professor of plant biology, began researching how to erase "allergen" genes in peanut plants as well as adding separate genes for disease resistance. Ultimately, the professor conceded in 2010 that given the number of proteins in peanuts, a hypoallergenic peanut was unrealistic.[47]

Legal systems were also challenged by the peanut-allergy epidemic. In 2000, the family of an Australian woman received a multimillion-dollar settlement from a restaurant after it had served her peanut-contaminated food. Her anaphylactic reaction had caused brain damage.[48]

In 2006, the Ontario provincial government passed Sabrina's Law, a nonpunitive expectation that all schools would comply with training, practices, and education in life-threatening allergies.[49] Between 2008 and 2010 the number of anaphylactic students in the Ontario public school system grew in just two years from 40,000 to 50,000. Their biographies with allergy profiles and photos decorated the walls of every teachers' lounge, ensuring that the entire community was aware of their status. Today most, if not all, Westernized countries have adopted policies on food allergy and its management in schools and child care centers. In 1999, the US courts confirmed that under the Americans with Disabilities Act, schools and day care centers must accommodate an individual's peanut allergy.[50] In 2006, the US government introduced the Food Allergy and Anaphylaxis

Management Act providing public K-12 schools with voluntary emergency guidelines.

While most people in the school community showed due concern for allergic kids, the "allergy bully" did not. Charges were laid in a groundbreaking 2008 felony case when a Kentucky eighth grader was accused of placing peanut butter cookie crumbs in the lunch box of another student.[51] And again in 2008, jail time was given to a nineteen-year-old Wenatchee, Washington, student who smeared peanut butter on the face of an allergic classmate.[52]

Despite the evidence, doctors still seemed polarized on the magnitude of the peanut-allergy problem. One doctor who pointed out that more people die from lightning strikes than from peanut called the peanut paranoia a mass psychogenic illness.[53] He referred to current behavior of parents and school staff as epidemic hysteria, citing the evacuation of a school bus full of ten-year-olds after a single peanut was spotted on the floor.[54] However, another doctor, exasperated British Member of Parliament Baroness Finlay of Llandaff called for increased funding for research and special allergy centers.[55] She was "extremely alarmed" about the Department of Health guidance given to pregnant mothers telling them to avoid peanuts. And yet, it was advice that Kate Middleton, Duchess of Cambridge, followed before becoming pregnant. In November 2011 the Duchess sparked rumors that she was already expecting when she refused a peanut paste snack others were eating during a visit to a UNICEF aid center. The palace would not comment except to confirm that Kate was not allergic to nuts.

At the end of the day, the questions "how and why is this happening?" were pushed to the side. What emerged instead in response to the apparent mystery was a massive food allergy industry, the infrastructure of which included billions of dollars in the sale of free-from foods, websites, blogs, magazines, parent-initiated lobby groups such as Food Allergy Initiative (est. 1998, www.faiusa.org) or the Anaphylaxis Campaign (est. 1994 in the United Kingdom), doctor-initiated associations such as Food and Allergy Anaphylaxis Network (est. 1991, www.foodallergy.org), and the many allergy and immunology associations for doctors and umbrella associations in Western countries such as the World Allergy Organization.

There was much overlap between the organizations, and all either created their own conferences or took part in annual trade shows that were, in turn, supported by fund-raisers, private donations, government grants, and pharmaceutical companies.[56] Pharmaceuticals—allergy drugs, testing, and medical research—made up an enormous part of the billions spent each year. Research in treatments for peanut allergy by 2014 included: oral immunotherapy (small doses of peanut flour to increase tolerance); peanut skin patch (patch with tiny teeth delivers small dose of peanut to increase tolerance); a vaccine that binds the 'allergy antibody' IgE with a virus so that the body will attack and destroy it; a prophylactic RNA vaccine for children who are *not allergic* (increases tolerance and induces IgG to block IgE); and a patented nine herbs FAHF formula (2005) for 'lessening' and helping to prevent peanut allergy. During 2004, 1,511,534 EpiPen prescriptions were filled in the United States representing 2,495,188 EpiPens.[57] By 2011, the US federal Bill S.1884 School Access to Emergency Epinephrine Act offered incentives to all states for the purchase of auto-injectors for their schools. The Bill offers that there are 6 million children at risk. Eventually, all 98,817 public schools will stock perhaps 100 of the devices annually. The potential gross sales if the devices are between $75 and $150 each is between $740 million and $1.48 billion each year. The companies likely to benefit from this Bill and Act are Mylan Inc. which sells EpiPens made by a subsidiary of Pfizer. They are in competition with Sanofi Aventis that makes Intelliject Auvi-Q a voiced-guided talking epinephrine injector. Registries such as Allergovigilance Network in France, the Food Allergy Register in Norway, and the ILSI European Food Allergy Task Force in Belgium began to collect data on anaphylactic reactions. EuroPrevall, a $14 million project, brought together over fifty-three research centers to investigate food allergy.

The WHO's Codex Alimentarius provided a handy top 8 list of "critical food allergens"—peanuts, tree nuts, dairy, egg, wheat, crustacean, fish, soybeans—and a downgraded list of 160 foods reported as able to provoke severe reactions. These lists and concomitant guidelines on their use in the food industry was a doubled-edged sword—useful on the one hand but invasive in the sense that the World Trade Organization (WTO) upheld WHO Codex Alimentarius guidelines in all trade disputes. This encouraged legislative change that forced manufacturers in many countries to comply with "guidelines." With the increasing reliance on and power given to WHO guidelines, it was proving problematic that the WHO had deemed it unnecessary to list, for example, refined peanut oil on food labels. This guideline extended to pharmaceutical labeling due to its GRAS (generally recognized as safe) status in the United States. Some pharmaceutical products—including vitamins, penicillin, and vaccines—historically have contained refined peanut oil and continued to include it without informing the consumer. Corporate law also shielded exact ingredients of patented pharmaceuticals.

With such intense activity and the proliferation of so much money, it was easy to lose sight of the presumed goal—unearthing the functional mechanism of sensitization—what was causing children to become sensitized to peanut in the first place? Again, the most significant clues were in the sudden emergence of the allergy just in children in specific countries and at the same time. But this obvious epidemiological information appeared nowhere in the flurry of papers that examined with mixed and often conflicting results the risk factors for developing peanut allergy.

Chapter 2

—◦∞◦—

RISK FACTORS

In successive waves through the 1990s, hundreds of thousands of peanut-allergic children arrived for kindergarten at public schools across the United States, Canada, Australia, the United Kingdom, and other Western countries. Critical mass, it seemed, was achieved almost overnight, catching educators off guard and prompting sudden changes in social behavior, shopping, and eating habits. Doctors had watched for years as prevalence of the allergy climbed and had become a special concern for children. With this unanticipated acceleration in children, a sense of urgency and desperation marked the medical literature until the early 2000s when research shifted to allergy treatments. Researchers analyzed any feature no matter how unlikely that seemed to distinguish peanut-allergic children from others.

Risk factors for the allergy such as atopy, maternal age, cesarean birth, socioeconomic status, and heredity ultimately were seen to contribute to allergic tendency; but none explained the specificity of the peanut or its sudden increased prevalence. Even geography was a misleading factor since it had been used as a convenient way to demarcate patterns of food consumption.[1] For this allergy, studies of peanut consumption and methods of peanut preparation and cultivation yielded few clues. Geography did hold significance but for a new pattern of toxicity seemingly specific to the Western lifestyle. A profile of the person most liable to develop a peanut allergy emerged from the known risk factors: a male child (male to female 2:1) born in a Westernized country after about 1990 whose ability to detoxify was challenged.

GEOGRAPHY

Geography was believed to be a primary risk factor for developing the allergy. An acknowledged but puzzling feature of the allergy was that it seemed to exist at first only in certain Western countries—the United Kingdom, parts of Europe, Canada, the United States, and Australia. Doctors were quite convinced that it simply did not exist in developing and Eastern countries such as China, India, or parts of Africa. In fact, explanations for the general rise in allergies such as the hygiene hypothesis rested on this East-versus-West observation. Starting in 2005, however, reports of peanut allergy in unexpected prevalence emerged from Hong Kong, Ghana, and Singapore. When word of these new outbreaks reached the medical community, the response was utter silence. No one could explain it.

The first reports regarding these new outbreaks indicated only serologic evidence with limited actual reactivity, but that quickly changed. By 2008, severe peanut reactions in children living in Hong Kong had increased: 1% of children aged two to seven were found to be reactive.

And in Cape Town, South Africa, again serologic evidence of peanut sensitivity was found in 5% of children studied in 2007 although reactivity was limited and nonanaphylactic. The reason for this hyporeactivity was already known. Helminths or intestinal worms dampened every immune reaction, and these children were heavily infested. However, by 2011 a study of Cape Town children with eczema found that peanut allergy was on the rise. The study concluded that the South African population had joined the food allergy epidemic widespread in Westernized countries. Similarly, a 2013 study reported that children 1.5% of children living in Ghana were reacting to peanut. This number was up from .53% in 2009.

And in Singapore, where peanut allergy in children was a "worrying trend" in 2007, by 2013 it had become a "common trigger" (see Appendix).

In fact, doctors had failed to notice a trend in the way the allergy suddenly emerged. A similar phenomenon had occurred in the United States. In 1994, 6% of the US population was reported to be sensitized to peanut although the vast majority was nonreactive. By 1997, 0.4% of American children under eighteen were reactive, but as in Hong Kong, this number quickly rose to 0.8% by 2002, to 1.4% by 2008 and in 2011 2% to 2.8% for children under 14 (see Appendix).

Taking this observation to a logical extreme, if sensitization grew at the same rate as documented reactivity in children, by 2002, 12% of the US population—about 35 million people—would be sensitized to peanut. In 2002, an estimated 1.04% of the US population was reactive to peanuts. Were the numbers then about 1:12? Meaning about three million actively peanut-allergic people for every 35 million sensitized? If that was true, whole populations were rapidly being sensitized somehow to their own food.

Using that modest percentage of 1.04% in 2002[2] for the top 5 countries, the total peanut-allergic population for 2002 was more than 4.3 million people: 3,057,600 in the United States; 327,704 in Canada; 613,600 in the United Kingdom; 92,332 in Sweden; and 205,165 in Australia. Although difficult to confirm, some believe this number in 2009 to have risen to an estimated 2% of these populations—7.36 million people.

Tracking the growth of peanut allergy from the start was a little like train spotting. Data was generated in small isolated studies that were then shared obsessively across the Internet and in medical journals. The upward trend in children continued to be monitored in the United Kingdom, the United States, and Australia, in particular. And yet in other countries—Norway, Denmark, Germany, and Japan—prevalence of the allergy was low (see appendix). In Estonia, Lithuania, and Russia, the allergy was of limited or no significance. And in sub-Saharan Africa and India, it seemed virtually nonexistent although this must be qualified by the paucity of studies and data available. The numbers of peanut-allergic children included the following:[3]

- 2.3% (2012) up from 1.71% (2007) for Canadian children
- 2% (2011) 1.4 % (2008) for US children
- 2% (2009) for UK children
- 0.45% or more (2002) for French children
- 1.2% to 2% (1999) or more (1998) for Swedish children
- 0.5% (2005) for Danish children
- .6% (2012) for Jewish Israeli children aged 13-14 which is up from .17% (2002). 2.5% (2012) for Arab Israeli 13-14 year old children
- 2.5% (2011) and another study 0.53% (2009) for Ghanaian children
- 1.11% (2009) for Australian children living in Tasmania
- 2% (2009) for Australian children living in the Australian Capital Territory
- 3% (2011) for Australian children living in Melbourne
- 1.08%–1.35% (2008) for Singaporean children
- 0.57%–1% (2009) for Chinese children living in Hong Kong

PEANUT CONSUMPTION

Ingestion of peanuts was originally believed to be a primary risk factor for developing the allergy. Researchers looked closely at methods by which peanuts were prepared, where they were grown, and levels and modes of exposure to them before and after birth. They were surprised to learn, ultimately, that the role of peanut consumption in the epidemic was anything but straightforward.

Boiling peanuts was thought to be the reason for the virtual nonexistence of the allergy in children living in China. This method of preparing peanuts reduced their allergenic proteins. Roasting, on the other hand, a common method of preparation in the United States, tended to enhance their allergenicity. However, using this observation to explain the lack of prevalence of the allergy in China proved difficult. Intact peanut proteins were still being consumed. As well, the allergy was not known to exist in India at this time where peanuts were prepared in a variety of ways, including roasted. As well, the emergence of the allergy in Hong Kong and Singapore, where boiling peanuts was ostensibly the preferred method of preparation, completely upended the idea. And finally, a 2010 study of 1 to 2 year olds from Chongqing, China, proved through oral challenge testing that food allergy had doubled between 1999 and 2009, from 3.5% to 7.7%.[4]

And farming methods and differences in soil were found to have no bearing on allergenicity of the peanut. Whether grown in Israel, India, or the United States, peanut proteins were the same.[5] Note has been made of the fact that peanuts also contain histamine and other substances that may affect allergenicity. Little research has yet been conducted on these in relation to proteins.[6]

And the common sense idea that eating a lot of peanuts contributed to the allergy was also problematic. In Sweden, where consumption of peanut was low, prevalence of the allergy in children was the same as it was in the United States.[7] The inverse was true for Jewish children living in Israel where peanut consumption was high and prevalence of the allergy was relatively low at .6%. And so, perplexed researchers turned next to analyze the allergic child and the tender age at which he or she first consumed peanut.

The most debated risk factor related to peanut consumption was whether consumption by pregnant and nursing mothers contributed to the prevalence of the allergy. Through the late 1990s, medical opinion on the issue swung from one extreme to the other—should mothers eat peanuts or stay away from them?—without consensus.

Some believed sensitization occurred in utero, before the child was born.[8] Others suggested it occurred during breastfeeding or through ingestion of refined peanut oil in baby formula. Some considered that since IgE antibodies do not cross the placenta, perhaps peanut proteins did and that perhaps fetuses swallowed IgE from amniotic fluid that then resulted in sensitization.[9] Doctors believed they had evidence from aborted fetal tissues showing that from the second trimester onward fetuses were capable of producing an allergic reaction. A French study of fifty-four infants who were less than eleven days of age and seventy-one who were seventeen days to four months of age found that 8% of the babies had a positive skin prick test for peanut.[10]

Another doctor urged that there was a lack of convincing evidence that manipulation of maternal diet during pregnancy had a lasting effect on the development of a food allergy. And therefore, it was thought lactation was a more likely route of primary sensitization.[11] Yet, another study in 2003 found no association at all between allergy and maternal peanut consumption while pregnant and breastfeeding.[12] Not content to leave the issue, further study in 2010 insisted that "maternal consumption of peanut during pregnancy is associated with peanut sensitization in atopic infants."[13]

A provocative university dissertation in 2007 determined that avoidance of peanut reduced the prevalence of the allergy but only in the child's first year of life.[14] Avoidance had no benefit after age one. The author Ting Liang admitted that this was difficult to explain. Liang suggested that there could be a "subtle" and as yet undiscovered environmental exposure to sensitizing proteins.

Ultimately, a worried British Department of Health issued a warning to pregnant and nursing mothers who had a history of atopy (other allergies) to avoid peanuts and all nuts to prevent peanut allergy. In 1998, the UK Committee on Toxicity of Chemicals in Food, Consumer Products, and the Environment issued a statement of avoidance.[15] The American Academy of Pediatrics also recommended delayed introduction of peanuts until three years of age for infants with a family history of allergies and maternal avoidance of peanuts during pregnancy and breastfeeding for mothers of such infants.[16] Observation that exposure to peanut oil hidden in vitamin supplements, nipple ointments, or soy formulae may contribute to sensitization was not rigorously examined. However, doctors had found some children were sensitized in this manner, and some even reacted.[17]

And yet, not only did this avoidance strategy have no effect on reducing prevalence of the allergy, but also it resulted in the highest number of peanut-allergic children yet seen in the United Kingdom.[18] One study put the number at 2.8% of children. A report to the UK parliament in 2007 concluded simply that this seemingly sensible government advice may have made things worse.[19]

And so, doctors made a complete about-face and asked whether it would be better for pregnant and nursing mothers to embrace peanuts and eat significant quantities of them. Exposure to peanuts during childhood was now thought to be crucial in developing immunological tolerance—it might even prevent the allergy. Conversely, a lack of peanuts could enhance sensitization.

A study in which English and Israeli children were compared concluded that the early introduction of peanuts in an Israeli food called *bamba* may have promoted tolerance and prevented peanut allergy.[20] In two populations of Jewish children ages four to eighteen in Tel Aviv and London, researchers looked at the roles of timing, frequency, and quantity of peanut consumption in the development of the allergy. The prevalence of the allergy was 1.85% in London and 0.17% in Israel in 2002. Among children ages four through twelve, the prevalence was 2.05% in England and 0.12% in Israel. When analysis was restricted to those at high risk for peanut allergy, those with confirmed eczema, the prevalence was 6.46% in England and 0.79% in Israel. By nine months of age, 69% of Israeli infants and 10% of English infants were eating peanuts. The main source was peanut butter made from roasted peanuts.

But if reduced exposure to peanut proteins led to allergy, then the protein-reduced boiled peanuts consumed in China should actually have created scores of peanut-allergic kids. The early introduction prevention theory made little sense especially in consideration of the prevalence of sesame allergy in Israel. Sesame allergy in Israeli children was almost as high as peanut allergy was in UK children. Ironically, Israeli studies claimed that the prevalence of sesame allergy in children was the result of their consumption of the food too early in life.[21]

Ultimately, the LEAP study (the Learning Early about Peanut Allergy study) emerged as a way to settle the issue of when and how to consume peanuts and to determine what was the best dietary strategy for prevention of the allergy.[22]

The much anticipated LEAP study published in February 2015[23] reiterated the theory of oral immunotherapy, what has been known for decades and what had been observed in Israel related to peanut allergy. The study indicated that early introduction and regular consumption of peanut in high risk children (those already with food allergy and/or eczema) resulted in a decreased risk of becoming reactive to peanut. But a discussion of what made the children high risk was not put forward. What caused the allergies and atopy that then made the children vulnerable to peanut and other serious food allergies?

To say that eating more peanut products regularly early in life solves the 'mystery' of the epidemic is to forget that peanut allergy became a societal concern only recently and suddenly in the early 1990s—prior to this time, ostensibly, we had been happily consuming peanuts in any amount without concern as to when or how.

One part of the LEAP study included 530 children aged 4 to 11 months of age with severe eczema, egg allergy or both who had had a negative skin-prick test result, no wheal, to peanut. From here, the children were randomly assigned to either avoid (limited exposure) or consume a baseline amount of peanut regularly for 60 months. It was determined that at 60 months of age 13.7% of the avoidance and 1.9% of the consumption group were allergic to peanut—as indicated by blood tests.

In both groups, IgE levels increased although it was higher in the peanut avoidance group. IgG was higher in the consumption group and wheals were smaller—all of this mirroring again what is known about oral immunotherapy, small doses of an allergen for some people may be consumed to reduce sensitivity. Whether the children retain this decreased sensitivity is not yet known. It was also suggested that exposure to peanut dust through the skin in children with eczema may contribute to sensitization. Peanut consumption was not possible at all for some children who were just too sensitive.

Again, the LEAP study was inspired by an observation that peanut consumption by children in Israel appeared to reduce prevalence of allergy. And yet, peanut allergy is on the rise in Israel.

In Israel, a study of adrenaline auto-injector dispensing rates from 1997 to 2004 showed a 78% increase.[24] According to the Israel Food Allergy Support Network (YAHEL) 8% of Israeli children now have serious food allergy. And topping the list of reactions according to ER hospitalizations in one Israeli hospital were nuts and milk.[25] By 2012, one study indicated that .6% of Jewish Israeli children aged 13-14 were allergic to peanut.[26] In 2002, that number was, again, .17%.

Allergy in children has been climbing so fast everywhere that despite the early consumption of any or all foods, the prevalence of anaphylaxis has and will continue to soar for the simple fact that no one is looking at causes. Treatments yes, but causes no.

The major clue to what is occurring in children, again, is found in the sudden development of anaphylaxis just in children, just in specific western countries and at the same time—no one knew that the children had become anaphylactic in such numbers until they showed up for kindergarten in the early 1990s.

There is only one functional mechanism of sensitization with the power to create this condition with such precision. The issue of when and how to consume peanuts was and is an expensive distraction.

In fact, a researcher on this team suggested that eating peanuts may not be the only method of sensitization: "The index allergic reaction usually occurs soon after the first known oral ingestion—which suggests that peanut sensitization does not always occur via the oral route."[27] Some doctors simply admitted that the exact route of primary sensitization was unknown although the gastrointestinal (GI) immune system was likely to play an important role.[28][29]

The GI system was long understood to play a significant role in allergies. For one, the successful catalytic effects of enzymes on proteins are crucial to limiting the movement of complete proteins into the bloodstream through the tissue of the bowel wall. A balance of specific microbes in the gut also helps maintain its integrity. With a compromised bowel, ill-digested proteins may be allowed to pass through and bind with blood serum, resulting in sensitization. As an explanation for epidemic anaphylaxis, however, scores of children would have had to experience bowel disease suddenly and at the same time in all the affected countries. In the extensive literature specifically on peanut allergy, there is no apparent investigation into a relationship with bowel disease. What would cause a sudden onset of bowel disease in children?

Allergist Kenneth Bock suggested in 2007 that low-grade infection in the GI tract possibly from vaccination would encourage allergic sensitization. Inflammation from such an infection sends out immune cell messengers that trigger even more inflammation in distant parts of the body. It can result in inflammation in joints, the lining of the GI tract, and even the brain. All inflammation, Bock suggested, contributes to allergies.[30]

In *Food Allergy: When Mucosal Immunity Goes Wrong*,[31] allergist Hugh Sampson suggests that the inflammatory bowel conditions such as celiac disease intersects with food allergy but may also reflect an IgE-mediated allergy to digestive flora. And inflammation of the gut may be accompanied by ongoing eosinophilic airways inflammation—this has been identified in peanut-allergic children.[32] At this juncture, two important question arise: did bowel inflammation and gut permeability lead to allergy? Or did the allergy develop first and lead to further inflammation? If it was the former, the search for a cause would have to start with a sudden onset of a gut condition in children starting around 1990, corresponding to the documented abrupt increase in peanut allergy in children at that time. If the latter then, again, there must be a specific mechanism of sensitization with the power to create allergy and atopy immediately and simultaneously just in children in specific westernized countries. This thought points directly at injection and vaccination the designed purpose of which is to provoke the immune system. But again, this is an area no one is willing to investigate. In fact, anecdotally, it has been banned in universities as an unwritten rule.

But as for simple consumption, in a 2007 report from the UK House of Lords, Science and Technology Committee confessed that levels and timing of consumption by mothers and children appeared to have an unclear relevance in the increasing prevalence of the allergy.[33] They offered that consumption of peanuts was up to individual discretion in consultation with a doctor. By 2010, the UK government advice was revised again—early-life exposure to peanut was no longer considered a risk factor for peanut allergy.[34] And finally, by 2015 the LEAP study raised questions about the "usefulness of deliberate avoidance of peanuts as a strategy to prevent allergy." The study suggests that timing and amount of peanut consumption contributes to lower risk of developing the allergy but should be consumed under the care of a doctor.

The act of eating peanuts as a mechanism for mass sensitization was at the least mired in conflicting information. At the worst, it was like seeing a tree but missing the forest. Mere consumption would not cause an epidemic of anaphylaxis in hundreds of thousands of healthy children, just in certain countries and with such abrupt prevalence. If atopy including eczema and other food allergies make one more vulnerable to developing peanut allergy, what was causing the atopy? The focus on a single mechanism of sensitization (eating or even peanut 'dust' through oozing skin) missed the probability that there was an additional and more powerful and specific determinant of creating allergy. In support, the specific and sudden rise of peanut allergy is a massive clue to understanding the big picture.

ATOPY: ECZEMA & ASTHMA

Atopy, from the Greek *atopos,* which means "out of place," is a medical term used to describe a tendency of an individual toward allergic conditions like eczema and asthma. Atopy that indicates increased levels of IgE antibodies is a generally accepted risk factor in the development of additional allergies.[35] Doctors were divided, however, on its relevance in the peanut allergy epidemic.

In a cohort study of American children referred for the evaluation of atopic dermatitis between 1990 and 1994, the prevalence of allergic reactivity to peanuts was nearly twice as high as that in a similar group evaluated between 1980 and 1984.[36] A 1996 study concluded that peanut allergy was rarely an isolated manifestation of atopy.[37] A Melbourne study of 620 atopic Australian infants in 1997 indicated that 1.9% were peanut allergic although egg (2%) and milk (3.2%) were more common at age two.[38]

In contrast, according to a 2006 study of Jewish children in Israel and the United Kingdom, the propensity to atopy did not explain the increasing prevalence of peanut allergy. Atopy was as prevalent in the UK children as those in Israel while peanut allergy was very low in Israel and high in the United Kingdom. Despite the study's unsteady conclusion that prevalence was related to a lack of early exposure (see "Peanut Consumption" above), it suggested that peanut allergy was independent of atopy. The allergy was seen in both supposed low-risk and high-risk children. The differences in peanut allergy could not, in this study, be explained by generalized differences in atopy.[39] The LEAP website indicates that just 20% of children with atopy (especially eczema or egg allergy) also developed peanut allergy. A 2011 study offered that food allergy has emerged as an unanticipated 'second wave' of the allergy epidemic in children, while asthma, rhinitis and eczema precede and predict food allergy. However, it was crucially important to point out that ISAAC (International Study of Asthma and Allergies in Childhood) that had compiled the data for the study did not include food allergy at its inception. Food allergy was considered more difficult to accurately determine and, therefore, ignored. This seems naturally to upend the idea that atopy preceded food allergy.[40]

But even if asthma and atopy were predictors for food allergy, what was causing the atopy? Was atopy genetic and independent of peanut allergy, or was there perhaps another underlying element that coincidentally linked both allergic conditions in children?

In 1997, one group of researchers thought they had found the connection. A Christchurch, New Zealand, longitudinal study followed 1,265 children born in 1977, twenty-three of which did not receive DPT and polio vaccinations. The nonvaccinated children had no recorded asthma episodes or consultation for asthma or other allergic illness before ten years of age. In the immunized children, 23.1% had asthma episodes, 22.5% asthma consultations, and 30% had consultations for other allergic illnesses. Similar differences were observed at ages five and sixteen years.

This study pointed to the pertussis toxin as having a direct IgE-inducing effect. Two other factors that promoted atopy in children were the aluminum-based vaccine adjuvants and the reduction in clinical infections in infancy.[41] In the process of building healthy immunity, the period from birth to six months of age was considered to be crucial. Some believed that certain vaccines had altered this process leading to atopy.[42] In fact, a retrospective study published in 2008 of Canadian children born in 1995 found that a delay in the DPT (whole cell pertussis) vaccination by 2 months was associated with a 50% reduction in asthma.[43]

At the same time, however, Japanese researchers saw an inverse association between tuberculin responses and atopic disorder: exposure and response to *Myobacterium tuberculosis* in a BCG vaccination appeared to inhibit atopic disorder through the lowering of serum IgE.[44] Ten years later, researchers found the opposite, stating that there was an absence of relationships between tuberculin responses and adult atopy and that the data was inconclusive.[45]

Doctors danced uncomfortably around the relationship of allergy and vaccination through the 1990s until finally the discussion was sidelined by a new and all-encompassing concept of allergy and immunity—the Th1/Th2 paradigm. This model of adaptive immune function argued that a balanced immune system could be disrupted by any number of factors, not just vaccination. Poor nutrition, vitamin supplements, parasite infection, lack of parasite infection, naturally acquired disease, or lack of disease could lead to atopy. The role of vaccination in atopy and allergy was thus engulfed by a massive construct that reduced it to just one of many immune-altering exposures.

BIRCH POLLEN ALLERGY

In Sweden, peanut consumption is low but the allergy to peanut is high. This being difficult to explain, researchers suggested that cross-sensitization to inhaled birch pollen was causing peanut allergy—this is known as 'oral allergy syndrome' or pollen-food allergy. A 2008 study of children in Sweden explained that the increase in allergy to peanut and tree nuts "probably reflects an increasing prevalence of allergy to birch pollen and pollen-related reactions to foods."[46] Researchers just weren't sure. And yet, even if it is assumed that the peanut allergy was caused by the birch pollen, how can the initial pollen allergy be explained in so many children and so suddenly, just in the last 20 years?

As early as 1959, researchers found that mice could be made severely allergic to grass pollen by using an adjuvant, an additive to provoke an immune response. In this instance, the mice were inoculated with a pertussis vaccine.[47]

A similar study took place in the late summer of 1973. Mice vaccinated again with a pertussis vaccine became sensitized to ragweed pollen that happened to be in the air at the time.[48] Subsequent intravenous injection of the mice with pollen extract resulted in an anaphylactic reaction. Creative researchers also found that they could create peanut allergy in mice through inhaled peanut if it was mixed with a toxic bacterium.[49] In these pollen-food or inhalation-ingestion experiments, again, a toxic adjuvant was needed to create allergy. This has yet to be investigated within the risk factor of pollen allergy.

TH1/TH2 PARADIGM DYSREGULATION

Doctors have religiously cited a general malfunction of the immune system as a risk factor for peanut allergy in children. The Th1/Th2 paradigm neatly organized the immune system by splitting it into two sides with two distinct thymus (T) white blood cell responses to pathogens and allergens. Doctors suggested that an upset in the balance between the two sides would almost certainly result in allergies. While it was a handy concept, the paradigm was later labeled as so much dogma unlikely to explain something as highly complex as the immune system. And as a risk factor in the epidemic, a dysregulation of the Th1/Th2 paradigm was not linked specifically to peanut allergy. It was just too broad.

White blood cells called T cells (matured in the thymus) and B cells (matured in bone marrow) circulate in the lymph, spleen, skin, and gastrointestinal tract where they react with antigens (i.e., bacteria, viruses). B cells proliferate and produce quantities of different antibodies, including IgE (immunoglobulin epsilon), the antibody most associated with atopy and allergy to deal with invaders that are outside the cells of the body (i.e., allergens). The B cells rely, in part, on information from T cells.

T cells deal with invaders that cause damage inside cells (i.e., viruses). They secrete cytokines (cell movers). There are two categories of T cells: cytotoxic T cells (killer T cells) that kill infected cells and helper T cells that enhance responses of other cells like macrophages and B cells. There are two types of helper T cells: Th1 and Th2. Th1 stimulates cell-mediated immunity. When Th1 cells recognize a viral antigen, for example, they secrete cytokines (interleukin 2 IL-2 and interferon IFM) to signal killer T cells to lyse or penetrate and destroy infected cells.

Th2 stimulate humoral immunity. When they recognize antigens, they produce cytokines (IL-4, 5, 10) that stimulate B cells to produce antibodies including IgE. The antibodies then bind to specialized IgE receptors on the surfaces of mast cells, basophils, and eosinophils in the bloodstream and connective tissue. These cells that contain allergy-inducing chemicals, such as histamine, are present in the connective tissues, in the respiratory tract, gastrointestinal tract, urinary tract, nasal passages, and skin. IgE antibodies can circulate in the bloodstream and become distributed on mast cells throughout the body. The allergic response begins when an allergen binds to IgE antibodies that are, in turn, bound to mast cells thereby activating the mast cells to degranulate and release their chemicals. Mast cell degranulation can result in vomiting, diarrhea, constriction of airways, coughing, sneezing, skin itch, a drop in blood pressure, and, in severe cases, shock and death.[50]

In the Th1/Th2 paradigm, a balance of the two T cell functions was seen as crucial. Nonatopic people show mainly Th1-immunity characteristics. They produce interferon that inhibits the growth of the Th2 cells. Again, some doctors suggested that vaccination was upsetting this balance by stimulating the Th2 side to produce excessive numbers of antibodies and limiting the Th1 (which would result in symptoms of disease).[51]

There was evidence that childhood infections (with fever and malaise) were important in the development of a balanced immune system by "teaching" the body how to handle other infections and that their vaccination-induced decline meant this developmental role was lacking.[52] And yet too much vitamin D,[53] some suggested, or genetic predisposition, could just as easily cause the imbalance.

By 2003, the paradigm that compressed the immune processes into a tidy concept itself came under fire. The "dogma that Th1 and Th2 cells are associated with cell mediated and humoral immunity, respectively, has recently been reevaluated . . . It appears that the mechanism of protection involves a complex combination of antibody and T-cell responses."[54] Such reevaluations suggested that antibody count—such as that of an IgE RAST test, as a measure of sensitivity to an allergen, or other antibodies, as a measure of vaccine efficacy—was just a small part of the total immune response.[55] The rigid model could not accommodate new data.[56]

AGE OF ONSET

The age of *onset* is the age at which the allergy is first discovered and not the moment of sensitization. Sensitization occurs before onset. Children born after 1990 carried a surprisingly increased risk of being both sensitized and reactive to peanut according to the Isle of Wight cohort studies, ER records, and eyewitness accounts as outlined in chapter 1. US studies indicated that prevalence of reactivity began to increase in those born between 1991 and 1997, and that by the year 2000, the percentage of children allergic to peanuts had surpassed the adult prevalence. By 2008, 1.4% of US children were peanut allergic.[57]

While the prevalence of the allergy in children climbed, the adult statistic remained relatively constant at about 0.5% of those over eighteen.[58] However, information pertaining to actual age of adult onset—age when those surveyed first discovered the peanut allergy—was not available as of 2010. An adult surveyed at age forty-nine (b. 1959) in the 2008 US phone survey, for example, may have developed peanut allergy after a heart attack and following the use of prescription drugs. This kind of information that would have helped pinpoint causes of peanut allergy was not included in the published US surveys.

As the numbers of allergic children climbed, the age of onset dropped. A review of pediatric peanut-allergic patients at Johns Hopkins University indicated a median age of peanut exposure and reaction were twenty-two and twenty-four months respectively for children born between 1995 and 1997; for those born before 2000, the ages were nineteen and twenty-one months; and for those born after 2000, their ages were twelve and fourteen months.[59] The ability to identify first exposure was anecdotal, using history and phone survey.

BIRTH MONTH

A correlation was discovered between the risk of developing severe allergy and the month of a child's birth. A study indicated that 55% of children born during

January through March had their first reactions to peanuts during those same months.[60] Similarly, 57% of children born in October through December experienced their first reactions during that three-month period. The same phenomenon was noted for those born between April and June. The correlation prompted speculation that dietary changes on or near a child's first birthday could explain the trend.

A Netherlands study detected an increased risk of cow-milk and egg allergies in patients born in November through January with a decrease in May. The same correlation was identified between period of birth and period of first peanut reaction.[61] In a study from Duke University, 31% of the peanut-allergic patients were born in October through December, compared with 18% in April through June. This leaves 51% born in July through September. This observation pointed to a possible relationship between environmental or seasonal factors, but lack of data prevented further speculation.

GENDER

The strong gender ratio difference in the peanut allergy went unnoticed by researchers until the later 2000s. Its significance was little understood but echoed the same striking trend in autism. Prevalence of peanut allergy was higher in boys than girls—in a ratio greater than 2:1.

Of 140 patients at a Duke University pediatrics clinic (70 born between 1988 and 1999, and 70 born between 2000 and 2005), 66% of those that were allergic to peanuts were male.[62] In a FAAN online survey, 67% of peanut-allergic children respondents were male. Similarly, of a Johns Hopkins University group, 63% were male.[63] Other studies supported this trend.[64] In an Australian ten-year survey of clinical consultation for food allergy in children under five, 60% were male.[65] A male predominance of peanut allergy was reported in children younger than eighteen years—1.7% versus 0.7% between males and females.[66] Only one study, a US CDC report from 2008, indicated that girls and boys were about even in prevalence of overall food allergy. While there was no explanation for the disparity between peanut-allergic boys and girls, a parallel phenomenon appeared in children with autism and Asperger's syndrome.

Hans Asperger, who identified the syndrome on the autism spectrum, originally believed that no girls were affected by the condition he described in

1944, although he later revised this conclusion. This gap was as high as 10:1 for Asperger's and 4:1 for autism. In 1964, Bernard Rimland observed that boys tended to be more vulnerable to "organic damage" than girls whether through hereditary disease, acquired infection, or other conditions.

The rate of autism and peanut allergy in children increased within the same window of time starting around 1990 with a concomitant gender ratio difference. The rate of autism in the United States was one in one thousand after 1970. Prevalence of autism spectrum disorders in the United States in 2006 was in the range of nine in one thousand children aged eight years[67] with an increase in those diagnosed starting in the late 1980s.[68] Peanut allergy had no significant profile prior to 1990. By 2009, it appeared in about one in seventy-five children in the United States and many other Western countries.

Increasingly, the health of boys and the birthrate of boys have been impacted by environmental pollutants at a higher rate than girls. The global decline in male births was nowhere more evident than in the Aamjiwnaang First Nations community in Ontario, Canada. In this small population down-river of polluting petrochemical plants, female births outnumbered male births 2:1 in 2003.[69]

RACE

Race was not seen to be a risk factor for developing peanut allergy.[70] However, geography, access to medical care, cultural norms, and socioeconomic and political factors can be associated with race. These factors may be reflected in the 2008 CDC National Health Interview Survey. In this survey, food allergy was reported in 3.1% of Hispanic children under eighteen years of age. This is significantly different from non-Hispanic white and non-Hispanic black children of whom 4.1% and 4% respectively had food allergies.

One study asked whether minority children were being underdiagnosed or undertreated for allergic conditions or whether they truly had a lower incidence of such allergies.[71] This 2005 study found significant racial, ethnic, and socioeconomic differences in the prevalence of childhood allergic disorders, especially peanut or tree nut allergy, but only as it related to prescribed injectable epinephrine.

Food-allergy reactions appeared to occur at a higher rate in Asian children living in Westernized countries.[72] One study found allergies in general to be higher in Asian than in European children in the United Kingdom.[73] In contrast, food allergy in Asian children living in China is traditionally low. Around 2005, however, this freedom from allergy changed when 1% of children living in Hong Kong were found to be peanut allergic and there was a doubling of food allergy in 1 to 2 year olds in Chongqing, China ~ from 3.5% in 1999 to 7.7% in 2009.

MODE OF DELIVERY AND INTESTINAL FLORA

Researchers suggested that a child born by cesarean section had an increased risk of developing allergies. They postulated that this mode of delivery used for one-third of US children delayed the growth of important flora in newborn intestine thereby impacting the immune system. Approximately 60% to 70% of the body's immune system is in the gut. While they conceded that cesarean was not linked to any specific allergy, it appeared to intensify atopy in general.

A Norwegian study focused on birth by cesarean section, the use of antibiotics in creating dysbiosis (bacteria imbalance in the digestive system), and low levels of digestive flora as risk factors in reactions to egg, fish, and nuts. Among the 2,803 children whose mothers were atopic, birth through caesarean section was associated with a sevenfold increased risk of reactions to foods. The association between caesarean and food allergy was not significant in children of nonatopic mothers nor was maternal or infant use of antibiotics.[74] These conclusions were echoed by a German study.[75]

Cesarean sections delayed the colonization of flora in newborn intestine. Balanced intestinal bacteria were seen as important for digestive health and the integrity of the colon. If ill-digested proteins managed to escape through the colon walls and enter the bloodstream, allergies could result. A subsequent article offered, however, that rather than increasing the overall risk of food allergy, cesarean simply made allergies worse.[76]

Yet another study from Finland found that allergic children had different fecal microflora with less lactobacilli and bifidobacteria. Probiotic and prebiotic supplements were given to 1,223 children over five years. Less IgE-associated atopy occurred in 24% of cesarean-delivered children who took the supplements.[77]

Cesarean births in the United States peaked at an average 24.7% of births in 1988 and then steadily declined between 1989 and 1996 before increasing yet again.[78] While the WHO recommended a maximum of 15% of births by cesarean, the US rate in 2006 was 31.1%.[79] In the United Kingdom, the cesarean birth rate was

10% in 1980, 11% in 1990, and 22% in 2002. In Israel, the cesarean birth rate was 10.7% in the 1980s,[80] 16% in 1999,[81] and 17–18% in 2006.[82]

While UK and Israeli cesarean rates were roughly comparable, prevalence of peanut allergy was significantly higher in the United Kingdom than in Israel (2% versus 0.17%, now increased to .6%). These figures were the inverse for sesame allergy in children. In Israel, 1.2% children were allergic to cow's milk and sesame, followed by egg (2002, 2008).[83] Sesame allergy in UK children in a 2005 study was low at 0.1%.[84] These significant differences cannot be explained by mode of delivery.

Cesarean birth like so many other factors appeared in general to exacerbate a tendency to allergy. But there was no specific link to the peanut allergy.

MATERNAL AGE AT DELIVERY

Since the average age of first-time mothers had gradually increased, doctors wondered whether it was a risk factor for allergy in children. As with many of the proffered general risk factors, it failed to shed light on the peanut allergy.

An American study of fifty-five severely food-allergic children sought to evaluate whether maternal age at birth was higher for children with IgE-mediated food allergy than for those without.[85] The mean maternal age at birth of children with food allergies was 31.2 years compared to the mean maternal age at birth of children without food allergies at 29.2 years. Mothers of children with a food allergy had 2.88 times greater odds of being aged above 30 years at the time of delivery compared to control patients: 78% compared to 55%.

While an explanation for this disparity was not ventured in the study, environmental factors may have contributed. According to the CDC statistics, there was a greater tendency for older mothers 30+ to have cesarean.[86] This mode of delivery was shown to exacerbate atopy in children born to atopic mothers. Again, though, there was no connection between maternal age and the puzzling features of the peanut allergy—including its epidemic acceleration after 1990.

SOCIOECONOMIC STATUS

The destruction of the Berlin Wall in 1989 and the fall of communism offered an opportunity for allergy researchers to better understand the divergent allergy trends in the two-halves of the city.

People in the less-affluent East Berlin had a significantly lower prevalence of atopic conditions than people living in the wealthier West. Within ten years of reunification, however, a study of children indicated that the two-halves had become the same in this regard. With reunification, researchers concluded, there came greater access to Westernized health care and lifestyle. Cleaning products, antibiotics, and other amenities had generally altered conditions for children born in the East and contributed to the increase in allergy, it was thought.

Between 2003 and 2006, the German Health Interview and Examination Survey for Children and Adolescents collected information on asthma, atopic dermatitis, hay fever, and eczema for 17,641 children aged one to seventeen. The survey revealed that there was increased sensitization to twenty common allergens.[87]

A loss of disease burden with improved socioeconomic conditions was presumed to have caused a dysregulation in the immune systems of children.[88] However, it seemed unlikely that in just ten years, East Berlin would have become sufficiently germ reduced and affluent to have prompted such a significant increase in atopy. This abrupt development suggested a more immediate and invasive cause.

Nevertheless, the Westernization of East Berlin did not explain the specificity of the peanut. In fact, prevalence of peanut allergy appeared to be low for children in Berlin, East and West.[89] In a randomly selected population-based survey of children in Berlin, the food allergens most commonly identified by oral challenge were apple, hazelnuts, soy, kiwi, carrot, and wheat. Food allergy symptoms, although no anaphylaxis, was shown in 4.2% of the children. All reactions were mild and mainly due to pollen cross-associated food allergy (oral allergy syndrome). In this study, peanut was not an issue. However, in a 2005 analysis of physician reported cases of 103 anaphylactic children in Germany, foods were the most frequent cause of the reaction (57% and 20% [eleven] to peanut of this number) followed by insect stings (13%) and immunotherapy injections (12%). Peanuts and tree nuts were the foods most frequently causing the reactions.[90]

The description of this risk factor, however, stopped short of delineating the specific features of socioeconomic status that were altered in East Berlin starting in 1989. The specific conditions that gave rise to peanut allergy elsewhere were presumably largely absent from East Berlin at this time. Given that the prevalence of the peanut allergy was still low ten years after reunification, those conditions may have continued to exist to some degree.

Other research noted a connection between socioeconomic status and prevalence of anaphylaxis in the United Kingdom.[91] Researchers used a map to highlight the more affluent areas of the country in which there was a slightly higher prevalence of anaphylaxis by virtue of ER admissions. Of these, reactions to drugs constituted over 50% of recorded triggers, and food made up almost 20%; children under five made up the majority of these patients. And yet, another UK study published in 2003 based on a longitudinal study in Avon saw no statistically significant associations between peanut allergy and any socioeconomic factor.[92]

LARGE HEAD CIRCUMFERENCE

Researchers in 1999 correlated the rise in allergy in children with the size of their heads. A study of newborn cord blood samples and measurements revealed an increase in IgE related to large head circumference.[93] IgE is traditionally thought to be produced only by the mother and cannot pass to the child. While this idea is being reviewed in the literature the level of IgE in the mother is thought to be a means of predicting a risk of future allergic tendency in the child.

The explanation for the relationship between a large head at birth and future allergy was curious. In affluent societies where nutrition is generally good, researchers explained, the fetus will grow rapidly during the early stages of pregnancy and will remain programmed to grow at this rate.[94] As the pregnancy progresses, the child will have a high nutrient demand, which is difficult to meet. In a poor community with poor nutrition, the fetus is programmed to grow slowly and have lower nutrient demand. The high-demand fetus is suddenly in a position where nutrient delivery is constant and therefore does not sustain growth. The brain and head continue to grow at the expense of the body that results in a big head and normal birth weight but poor nutrient delivery to other parts of the body. This, in turn, modifies the immune system. Apparently, the Th1 side is more susceptible to being switched off in adverse circumstances than Th2. Thus, it was suggested, the relationship of a large head and suppressed Th1 side explained the increase in allergy in affluent societies.

While having a large head at birth may point to future allergies, according to limited studies, it did not explain the sudden accelerated prevalence of peanut allergy starting around 1990.

HEREDITY

A broadly accepted risk factor in the development of allergy in children is heredity. While statistics revealed common allergy threads between siblings and mothers, again, this risk did not fit with the simple facts of the peanut allergy—its abrupt emergence around 1990 and its rapid spread. Genes do not change that quickly.

In 1996, it was observed that peanut allergy was more common in siblings of people with peanut allergy than in the parents or the general population.[95] The higher rate of peanut allergy in the siblings of people with peanut allergy compared with the general population was about 7% versus 1.3% in one study.[96] Peanut allergy was reported by 0.1% (3 out of 2,409) of grandparents, 0.6% (7 out of 1,213) of aunts and uncles, 1.6% (19 out of 1,218) of parents,[97] and 6.9% (42 out of 610) of siblings according to a 1996 study.[98] In 2000, one researcher performed a study of monozygotic and dizygotic twins aged one to fifty-eight in which one of the pair had the peanut allergy. Skin tests performed suggested that because more nonreactive monozygotic pairs had a positive test, than dizygotic pairs that there was a genetic influence on peanut allergy.[99]

This study defaulted to the idea that there may be an "allergy gene" that condemned some families to allergy.[100] It avoided discussion of differences between the twins as individuals with different medical experiences, gender, history, digestive health, kidney function, and abilities to detoxify waste.

The same differences may have been at play in a provocative study using different strains of genetically engineered mice. The study showed that injections of peanut-induced anaphylaxis in some but not all strains.[101] After vaccination with peanut, the mice were injected again three or five weeks later. Researchers were unable to induce anaphylaxis in two strains of albino mice AKR/J and BALB/c—neither IgE or IgG1 were found in these two strains although IgG2a was increased. Anaphylaxis was easily induced in the gray-brown C3H/HeSn strain. A general genetic explanation was offered for these differences that, researchers proposed, might also exist in humans.

This vision of DNA was formulated by Francis Crick who, together with James Watson, deciphered the structure of the DNA molecule in 1953. Crick came to believe that DNA controls life, a ubiquitous concept that is usually accepted as incontrovertible fact.

While moderate doctors such as Kenneth Bock suggested "genetics may load the gun but environment pulls the trigger,"[102] a new generation of scientists has rejected the Crick DNA dogma outright. Genetics did not load the gun, the environment did under the new concept of epigenetics.

Cell biologist Dr. Bruce Lipton in his research at Stanford University School of Medicine in the early 1990s suggested that the environment, operating energetically through the membrane of the cells, actually controls the behavior and physiology of cells. In other words, the human body is not a biochemical machine at the mercy of self-actualizing genes (turn themselves on and off), but rather environment and the individual's perception of it control gene activity. Cells possess the ability to reprogram their own DNA as they are affected by diet, chronic thoughts, and even vaccination. Such rewriting accounts for up to 98% of evolutionary transformation. In short, epigenetics suggested that people are masters of their own biology. If this were true, there would be implications for a broader understanding of peanut allergy and perhaps also how to recover from it.

The traditional understanding of genetics, however, cannot explain the peanut allergy epidemic. Hundreds of thousands of children would have had to experience a simultaneous change in their genetic profile starting around 1990 and occurring regularly and increasingly since then to account for the current peanut-allergy phenomenon. This would have been highly unlikely.

IMMUNE SYSTEM OVERLOAD

The four As—allergy, autism, ADHD, and asthma—have emerged from fundamental dysfunctions in nutritional, immune, and inflammatory factors, suggested Ken Bock in *Healing the New Childhood Epidemics* (2007).[103] Contributing to these unhealthy conditions in many children were the following: fungal overgrowth, especially candida that has spread from the gut; poor diet and eating habits; and deficiencies in probiotics (beneficial digestive flora), essential fatty acids, stomach acid, and digestive enzymes. Further crippling a child's immune system were antibiotic overuse and childhood vaccinations.

If a robust Th1-side immune response is not established, Bock offered, a child can develop a chronic low-grade infection from an injected vaccine antigen, such as measles. Such an infection can linger in the gut resulting in inflammation, which in turn sends out immune cell messengers, cytokines, that trigger even more inflammation in distant parts of the body. This can lead to inflammation in joints, the lining of the gastrointestinal tract, and even the brain. All inflammation contributes to allergies, stated Bock. And allergies cause even more inflammation.

While these overlapping factors contributed to the prevalence of the four As, the smoking gun that explained the sudden prevalence of peanut allergy had yet to be unearthed.

VACCINATION

Bock (2007) pointed to the mercury preservative thimerosal in vaccines as a significant factor in the epidemics of autism, ADHD, asthma, and allergies in children. He also expressed concern over the increase in the number of vaccines, the multidose single shots, unidentified health conditions of the child at the time of vaccination, and more.[104]

For scientists, it was difficult to confirm the role of vaccination because there were no studies of nonvaccinated populations in the United States—there were so few children who had not been vaccinated. According to the CDC, US vaccination rates have been at record highs. While 77% of US kids met all vaccination goals in 2007, at least 90% met the goal for each vaccine except for DTaP, but even those kids received three out of the four recommended doses.[105]

Recognizing that there was a significant gap in medicine's understanding of vaccination outcomes, two members of the US Congress introduced the Comprehensive Comparative Study of Vaccinated and Unvaccinated Populations Act in 2007. This bill was slow to achieve support and was reintroduced to the 111th Congress in 2009.[106]

In 2007, a grade 9 Connecticut student Devi Lockwood[107] conducted an ad hoc study of the few nonvaccinated populations in the United States. Devi looked at the Old Order Amish who discouraged vaccination. In these communities, peanut allergy was virtually nonexistent. But because the Amish communities were genetically connected, their example in understanding the role of vaccination in allergy was rejected by the CDC.[108]

And so, Devi turned to Vashon Island, Washington, a haven for alternative medicine where 1,600 school-aged children were unvaccinated. Devi looked at two schools, elementary and middle, with high exemption rates on Vashon Island and two similar schools in his hometown of Ridgefield that had low-exemption rates. Where the vaccination rate was high, the prevalence of peanut allergy increased significantly. Where vaccination rate was low, so, too, was the prevalence of the allergy. At the two Vashon schools, there were three peanut-allergic children. In Ridgefield, there were twenty-two at the two schools. All peanut-allergic children had been vaccinated. Significantly, there were no unvaccinated children with peanut allergy in this small study.

Risks associated with vaccination were infrequently ventured in medical literature through the 1990s although increasing in the later 2000s. Vaccination, an event shared by the vast majority of Western children, carried clear political, social, and economic implications. Doctors would not or could not dissuade the public from getting their shots. And yet, the connection between allergy and vaccination was not new—the literature was clear about the allergencity of vaccines and even provided an example of a causal role in the outbreak of gelatin allergy in children starting in 1994. The relationship between injection and allergy has long been established (see chapter 4) and as the potency of adjuvanted vaccines increased through the 1970s researchers warned "that the regular application of aluminium compound-containing vaccines on the entire population could be one of the factors leading to the observed increase of allergic diseases."[109] And yet, vaccination is largely absent from the plethora of research on peanut allergy. As already noted, as a potential means of causing atopy, vaccination was lumped together with every other risk factor within the broad shouldered hygiene hypothesis (See chapter 3).

EAR INFECTIONS, ANTIBIOTICS & GUT FLORA

Children receive an average of 2.2 antibiotic prescriptions in the first year of life according to a 2013 study.[110] The study looked at two groups of children born between 2007 and 2009—those diagnosed with food allergies and those without. In this study, children who had had 2.65 antibiotic exposures compared to 1.84 exposures were at greater risk for food allergies as measured by IgE antibodies.

The study speculated on the destructive impact antibiotics have on digestive flora and how this might contribute to allergies.

In 2014, a study of mice from the University of Chicago Medical Center indicated that Clostridia, a common gut bacteria, reduced allergic sensitization. In the study, mice were treated with antibiotics then force-fed peanut thereby inducing a rise in IgE antibodies against the peanut. By re-introducing Clostridia to their digestive tracts the mice experienced a reduction antibodies specific to the peanut. According to study authors, "Clostridia caused innate immune cells to produce high levels of interleukin-22 (IL-22), a signaling molecule known to decrease the permeability of the intestinal lining."[111]

It is important to note that none of the mice actually reacted to peanut. Rather, antibodies found in blood work indicated sensitization.

These findings support the 'Expanded Hygiene Hypothesis' (see chapter 3) which implicates pharmaceuticals in the general rise in allergies.

But why are children being given such quantities of antibiotics in their first year of life? Ear and throat bacterial infections, often strep, are common reasons for antibiotic use in children.

Between 1988 and 1994, there was a significant increase in ear infections among US children.[112] In this time frame, the number of children with ear infections under one year of age went up by 3 percent and recurrent ear infections (3 or more) increased by 6 percent—this latter figure representing an increase of 720,000 more children in the 6-year period.

But what was causing this soaring number of infections for which antibiotics were prescribed? Many doctors and naturopaths point to back undiagnosed food allergies.

In a 1994 *Annals of Allergy* study, 86% of children had a significant reduction in ear infections simply by eliminating allergenic foods from their diet (wheat, eggs, corn, etc.).[113] Another study showed that children allergic to cow's milk were twice as likely to have recurrent ear infections. This allergy often goes undiagnosed although the relationship between dairy allergy and ear infections has been known for decades. A respiratory imbalance caused by dairy allergy known as Heiner syndrome causes recurring ear infections. Dr. David Hurst specializing in ENT has dedicated a web site to the role of allergy in ear infections stating that "allergy is the cause of most chronic middle ear fluid, and that aggressive use of standardized allergy management can solve the problem:"

It is my contention that the middle ear behaves like the rest of the respiratory tract and that what has been learned about the allergic response in the sinuses and lungs may be applied to the study of the ear to help in understanding the pathophysiology of chronic otitis media with effusion (OME).[114]

Again, if the root cause of ear infection is food or environmental allergies that in turn causes inflammation and fluid that invites infection for which antibiotics are required (causing more allergies) *what caused those initial allergies?*

This appears to be a circular discussion. However, one might suspect that while antibiotics make one more vulnerable to allergies, there is yet another sensitizing mechanism at play such as vaccination which is a well known cause of allergy and anaphylaxis. With vaccination the goal of immunity and allergy are inseparable—both defenses are provoked simultaneously.

GENETICALLY MODIFIED FOODS & HERBICIDES

The safety of genetically modified foods has been a significant concern since the 1980s.

Concern regarding the transfer of allergens from one plant or seed to another without informing the consumer emerged in the 1990s. For example, when genes from brazil nuts were used to enhance soybeans allergy experts objected. Guidelines rather than regulations seemed to apply but common sense ruled the day after testing patients allergic to brazil nuts with the soybean. The risk of reactivity through GMOs to those allergic was no longer theoretical.[115]

There was also a risk for the creation of allergies to previously unknown genetically engineered proteins (whether consumed directly or through gene transfer via animals fed the GM plants). These proteins new to humans are cause for concern but there has been no specific evidence linking them to a rise in allergy much less the sudden documented rise around 1990.

GM 'roundup ready' soybean by Monsanto was approved for growth in the US in 1995. The 'roundup ready' gene made the soybeans resistant to Monsanto's Roundup herbicide known as glyphosate—this gene allowed farmers to spray the herbicide on the engineered soybean crops to kill surrounding weeds without harming the soybean plants.

Roundup/glyphosate was first introduced to farmers in 1974. The herbicide inhibits an enzyme 'shikimate' pathway in normal plants. This pathway synthesizes (makes available) essential amino acids tyrosine, tryptophan and phenylalanine. These amino acids are called 'essential' because humans need them to live and are unable to produce them without plants and bacteria. Again, glyphosate/roundup disrupts the shikimate pathway and kills plants that are not 'roundup ready' ie. the 'weeds.'

In this process of 'improving' crops it was assumed that humans who do not have a shikimate enzyme pathway would not be impacted by the herbicide. It turns out, however, that common bacteria in the human digestive tract do have this pathway and that glyphosate interferes with their synthesis of these amino acids. And so, consuming this herbicide via soybean in processed foods, for example, would disrupt our gut microbiome and reduce the availability of these amino acids. Additional studies conducted by Dr. Stephanie Seneff of MIT indicates that the impact of this herbicide also impairs sulfate transport and other enzymes crucial in our abilities to detoxify.

While the disruptive role of herbicides is clear, that of GM foods is not. Certainly, as discussed in the section on antibiotics the loss of certain bacteria has impacted the integrity of the small intestine. Glyphosate no less contributes to this loss and 'leaky' gut which can lead to food sensitization and a rise in IgE.

However, neither the consumption of herbicides which has been constant nor GM foods correlates with the epidemiological facts of the peanut allergy epidemic. The sudden phenomenon of this allergy as it emerged just in children, only in specific countries and at the same time 1988 through 1994 is too abrupt, too precise a development to be explained by herbicide exposure that had been constant for decades or the gradual increasing consumption of GM foods.

THE NOCEBO EFFECT & OWNING YOUR BODY

The word placebo was first used in a medical context by British physician William Cullen (1710-1790). In his 1772 lectures, Cullen described the use of a remedy for an incurable case in order to bring comfort and 'please' the patient. Cullen was a follower of 'sympathy' or 'vitalism' and coined the word 'neurosis' suggesting in *First Lines in the Practice of Physick* (1790) that "almost all diseases considered on a certain point of view could be considered nervous". Our current meaning of placebo in drug experiments, for example, compares subjects given an active drug with others given a sham or placeco substance (sugar pill). When those receiving the sugar pills experience positive effects or were 'pleased' by the placebo it is suggested that the subject's mind or positive belief caused the improvement.

In contrast, the nocebo reaction mentioned first in 1961 by physician Walter Kennedy is one in which a negative belief causes negative physical symptoms. The nocebo effect has been documented many times. In a study of drug allergic patients 27% of those allergic reacted to an inert substance believing it was the drug to which they were allergic.[116] While it seems clear that one's expectation and beliefs are linked to reactivity it is tantalizing to speculate on how belief might contribute to initial sensitization.

A 2011 study showed that what one believes about one's own body can contribute to an 'up-regulated' immune response.[117] In an experiment at the University of South Australia, a team of neuroscientists discovered that if one has a 'lost sense of ownership' over a part of their body or even the entire body, the body will reject it to some degree (part or all) with a corresponding intense up-regulated immune response. In their experiment, the team injected hista-mine into the arms of volunteers while they were under the false impression that one of their arms had been substituted with a rubber arm. The immune response at the 'replaced' or 'disowned' arm was consistently and significantly bigger.

Lead researcher Lorimer Moseley was quoted in *Science Alert* (Jan. 2012):

"These findings strengthen the argument that the brain exerts some kind of control over specific body parts according to how strongly we own them."

"OUTGROWING" PEANUT ALLERGY

No one knew how or why a child "outgrew" a peanut allergy. And even when a child did, this resolution of the allergy was not always permanent. Statistics reported in 2001 indicated that as many as 22% of peanut-allergic children developed tolerance to the food later in life.[118] Chances of outgrowing the allergy were improved if the child had low levels of peanut-specific serum IgE antibodies in infancy (less than 5kU per liter).[119]

A 1998 study of fifteen children compared those who had outgrown their clinical reactivity to peanut and those who had not. All children "resolvers" and "persisters" had reacted to peanut first at the age of about eleven months, and they were retested at about age five.

Although in skin prick tests, resolvers had much smaller wheals, blood tests showed that the IgE total and peanut-specific levels between the two groups did not differ.[120] Allergy to other foods was less common in resolvers (2 of 15) than persisters (9 of 15).

In a phone follow-up two years later with the resolvers in this study, only one had reacted by vomiting after eating peanut. A note of caution no doubt accompanied the news of this apparent resolution, however, since some children previously thought to have outgrown the allergy have reverted.[121]

An unusual case was reported in 2005 of a child whose peanut allergy resolved following a bone marrow transplant.[122] In this instance, not only was a food challenge negative, but also specific IgE to peanut was found to be undetectable (<0.35 KU A).

SUMMARY OF RISK FACTORS

The frantic attempts to find common ground between the hundreds of thousands of peanut-allergic children as the 1990s unfolded revealed a profound level of confusion. Intense study had been made into peanut consumption, the role of atopy, and other possible risks leaving researchers with more questions than answers. And despite the preponderance of research, significant risk factors such as gender, bowel condition, and vaccination were given little or no attention.

Deepening the concern of perplexed doctors was the unanticipated appearance of the allergy in China and Africa through the 2000s. Many had bet their reputations on the idea that just eating peanuts was a primary risk for developing the allergy and that boiling peanuts had protected the Chinese from it.

What emerged from the tangle of research ultimately was a partial profile of the person most at risk for developing the allergy: a child (male 2:1) born after 1990 in a Westernized country and whose ability to detoxify had been challenged by environmental factors. These factors appeared to include vaccination, but such a proposal amounted to a hypothesis very much at odds with official medical explanations for the phenomenal rise in allergy in the twentieth century.

Chapter 3

---❦---

THEORIES

By 2000, doctors had matched general risk factors with clinical observations to produce several explanations for the general rise in allergy. Each disparate theory, however, was a bad fit for the peanut allergy. None could adequately explain its sudden and increased prevalence initially only in children living in certain Western countries.

Theories applied to the peanut allergy included the broken-skin hypothesis, the ingestion hypothesis, the helminth hypothesis, the hygiene hypothesis and the expanded hygiene hypothesis. Fundamental to each of these was a definition of allergy as a "genetically determined disorder."[1] Each assumed that allergy is an inherited dysregulation of the immune system that leads to an elevated production of IgE antibodies in response to protein allergens.[2] And as such, if the environment contributes to a child's allergy, it merely unmasks an extant predisposition to reactivity. Genetics loads the gun, and the environment fires it. Humans are fated to allergy.

The toxin hypothesis, developed before the peanut-allergy epidemic emerged, provided a lone counterpoint to the official hypotheses. This hypothesis was alone in its proposal that allergy is not a dysfunction at all. Within this new concept, allergy serves a purpose as an evolved immune defense against acute toxicity. Whether sensitized to toxic proteins by inhalation, broken skin, injection, or consumption, the purpose of the allergic response is to eject the toxic threat from the body as fast as possible. The idea that this dangerous reaction may have a designed purpose was an important clue that doctors had either missed or dismissed.

Indeed, at the end of the day, a kind of medical myopia appeared to constrain the perspective of many researchers. Few were motivated to look for clues outside of the immediate specimens of child or peanut proteins. American microbiologist René Dubos had observed that it is seldom recognized that each society and every civilization creates its own diseases.[3] If this was true, then a broad framework of investigation that embraced other areas of thought, including history, could be required to drag the solution into public consciousness.

BROKEN-SKIN HYPOTHESIS

It was proposed in a 2003 study that exposure to low doses of peanut proteins through broken and inflamed skin had caused mass allergic sensitization to the food in children.[4] Researchers were surprised to find that many eczema ointments commonly used on children contained refined peanut oil. An analysis of the oil revealed that there were enough intact proteins to sensitize atopic children to peanuts. This, they suggested, was the source of the epidemic.

Data was used from the Avon Longitudinal Study of Parents and Children, a geographically defined cohort study in southwest England of 13,971 preschool children. In this group, there were 49 children confirmed to have peanut allergy. Questionnaires, medical records, biologic samples—including cord blood which in containing IgE is traditionally thought to have been produced by the mother and not passed to the child—provided information on children born in 1991 and 1992 up to the age of about three years. Of significance was their belief that sensitization to peanut occurred after birth.

To explain the allergy to peanuts, researchers developed a somewhat complex theory based on two risk factors. The first was that there was a strong association between eczema caused by an intolerance to cow's milk and peanut allergy. Although none asked what had caused the milk allergy, it was a problem because mothers then switched their children from milk to a soy beverage. This decision became the real risk factor, they argued, because it could have sensitized the children to soy proteins that are similar to those of peanut. Significantly, none of the peanut-allergic children in this study appeared to be reactive to soy—they could consume it without apparent concern. However, this phenomenon was not unusual. In a 2002 article, allergist Hugh Sampson pointed out that while most patients with peanut allergy do have IgE antibodies against other legume proteins,[5] fewer than 15% of these people react to them. Furthermore, any reaction to other legumes tended to be less severe, and these allergies were rarely lifelong.

Once sensitized ostensibly to soybean in this hypothesis, peanut entered the scenario via a second risk factor—refined peanut oil in skin ointments[6] that were applied to the skin that was broken and inflamed with eczema (dairy must then not have been the only cause of eczema because it had been removed from the diet).

The oil in the skin ointments was alleged to be free of sensitizing peanut protein. However, researchers analyzed the oil and found that it contained enough protein to produce "positive responses in leukocyte histamine-release assays in such patients."[7] Additional studies in 2005 supported this idea concluding that epicutaneous exposure to peanut protein could cause oral intolerance in experiments with mice.[8] And yet, an equal number of atopic children with eczema did not develop peanut allergy. This gave rise to doubts that therapeutic pharmaceutical products containing refined peanut oil played a role in sensitization.[9]

Scanning back in time, crude peanut oil loaded with the dangerous proteins had been used on skin with cuts and abrasions for decades without apparent incident. The health benefits of rubbing peanut oil on skin were recommended by agricultural chemist George Washington Carver (1864–1943) to help heal polio. Carver was certain that peanut oil applied during a massage not only saturated the skin and flesh but also actually entered the bloodstream and helped restore life to limbs withered by polio. In 1933, the Associated Press carried a story about Carver's alleged successes with polio peanut oil massages, and for a time, his Alabama school resembled a pilgrimage site. Thousands of Americans, including President Franklin D. Roosevelt who visited Carver in 1938, enjoyed a peanut oil rubdown. Doctors recommended and developed their own brand such as the Vitalized Peanut Oil in 1934.[10] Not to be outdone, another skin oil entrepreneur, the Rose Miller Company, sought approval from the FDA for its peanut oil "bust developer."[11]

Indeed, peanut oil in ointments for eczema and other skin conditions had been constant for decades. There was no sudden acceleration of use that would have coincided with the abrupt increase of peanut-allergic children starting around 1990. The broken-skin hypothesis did not include an explanation for this event.

The use of peanut oil, refined or not, in skin creams does not explain the sudden and continuing rise of this allergy in children. It does, however, open questions on the use of refined peanut oil or other cross-reactive legume oils such as castor bean oil or soybean oil in other potential methods of sensitization such as oral or injected pharmaceuticals.

The relative allergenicity of refined peanut oil did not worry the US Food and Drug Administration, however. The FDA had given refined peanut oil GRAS (generally recognized as safe) status. GRAS indicates that its use in food is presumed safe based either on a history of use before 1958 or on published scientific evidence. A manufacturer does not need approval by the FDA to use the oil in foods.[12] And yet, in 1998, researchers confirmed that refined peanut oil did contain trace proteins that were the same as those in crude peanut oil.[13] The FDA at their website acknowledged the studies and observed that the levels of peanut protein varied due to differences in refining processes and the detection method used. According to this agency, "most highly refined oils contained 0.2–2.2 µg/ml of protein."[14] But again, it was not a concern.

Nut and seed oil refiners Welch, Holme & Clark Co. published a webpage on "Refined Peanut Oil NF."[15] "NF" stands for *national formulary* from the US Pharmacopeia (USP). The NF is a book of public pharmacopeial standards for medicines, excipients, and other mixtures. In it is a procedure for refining peanut oil.[16] According to the Welch, Holme & Clark site, "high-quality" peanut oil is extremely difficult to obtain because almost all refined peanut oil contains traces of cottonseed oil—even in small quantities the presence of cottonseed oil violates the specifications of the USP.

Including a "high-quality" refined peanut oil implied that there were those of low quality. To that end, the WHO Codex Alimentarius Committee on Food Labeling resisted giving its full endorsement to the oil in 2000.[17] While DBPC tests in which peanut allergic volunteers consumed refined peanut oil without reaction, the WHO questioned the refining processes and lack of thorough data and even the quality and validity of the analytical procedures used to determine the concentration of residual protein in the oils.

Ultimately, instead of investigating the allergenicity of the oil further, the WHO committee relied on the oil's history of previous use and made no decision regarding the inclusion of refined peanut oil in foods on labels.[18] There were two allergenic foods of debate that may or may not be labeled: refined peanut oil and refined soyabean oil. Based on the US Food Allergen Labeling and Consumer Protection Act of 2004, Sec. 203, subsection 7, part C.c.1.qq.2.1 under Conforming Amendments, highly refined oils are exempted as major food allergens and exempted from labeling. In US-made foods, refined peanut oil was still not labeled in 2009.

And yet, children have been sensitized to refined peanut oil contained in oral vitamin D supplements.[19] And the peanut oil used in baby formula had caused anaphylaxis in infants sensitized to peanut.[20] Some doctors argued that peanut oil should be excluded from medications altogether or at least listed as an ingredient.[21]

While doctors remained divided on the allergenicity of refined legume or nut oils in foods, skin creams, and oral medications, it seemed beyond the bounds of discussion to review their inclusion in injected products.

If researchers in the broken-skin hypothesis were suspicious of the cross-sensitizing properties of refined soybean oil in baby formula, surely they would be concerned that it (as lecithin E322) and another legume oil, castor bean, were ingredients in popular brands of the injected vitamin K1 prophylaxis. In Western countries, virtually all children receive the vitamin K1 injection within moments of birth.

And the refined peanut oil described for use in foods that had sensitized some children was the same oil used in some medical injections. At the Welch, Holme & Clark website was a declaration that their refined peanut oil "fully meets USP specifications in every respect and is suitable for injectable use."[22] As of 2010, there were no apparent published investigations into this potential route of sensitization despite the fact that it was common to all children.

Another proposed risk for sensitization to peanut was skin prick testing (SPT) or scratch testing used by allergists in diagnosing allergy. In this test, a drop of diluted allergen is placed on the skin that is then pricked with a pin. A wheal will form at the wound that is supposed to indicate a patient's level of sensitivity. However, this test has come under fire for accuracy, false positives and actually creating allergy according to anecdotal evidence. In "Skin Testing in the Diagnosis of Food Allergy, limitations and risks" (2004) Canadian Dr. Janice Joneja suggests that this test is not harmless but rather demonstrates that an immunological response has occurred. In support of the real possibility of sensitizing via the SPT, she points to 'patch' immunotherapies that deliver tiny doses of allergens in a patch worn on the arm. Little to no research has been conducted on the possibility of sensitization via SPT. However, again, the sudden and increased prevalence at the same time in the same countries still begs the question of a profound and initial functional mechanism of sensitization that would then, secondarily, necessitate allergy testing and SPT.

INGESTION HYPOTHESIS

Researchers seemed to think that by pinpointing how and when children first ate peanut, they could solve the epidemic. It was presumed that just eating peanut could result in sensitization if a child had a compromised digestive system. Alternatively, genetics contributed to sensitization if the child had an inherent dysregulation of the Th1/Th2 paradigm. In this hypothesis, though, there was no specific mechanism of sensitization to peanut. The allergic individual was assumed to have a tendency to capricious sensitization. And the fact that peanut was so allergenic only increased the chances of becoming sensitized to it.

While the theory of ingestion was obvious and easy to comprehend, as an explanation for an epidemic of food allergy, it did not fit. Although allergists have stated that "ostensibly, ingestion of peanut is the sensitizing route,"[23] this risk factor was fraught with conflicting data and confusion. As reviewed in chapter 2, many studies indicated that ingestion of peanut—early or later in life, boiled, roasted or refined, in breast milk or nipple creams, in small or large quantities—had an unclear relevance in the rapid rise of this allergy in children.

It was difficult to accept that hundreds of thousands of children had become allergic to this one food in the space of just twenty years by ingestion alone. The hypothesis proposed that all peanut-allergic children (an average of 58,000 US children a year between 1997 and 2002 reaching 580,000 peanut-allergic children under eighteen in 2002[24] and 1,000,000 by 2008) had weakened digestive abilities or a Th2 skewed system, or both. The large numbers alone were just too great to sustain such an explanation unless there was indeed a mechanism that had caused the GI tracts of these children to somehow fail at the same time. There has been no apparent inquiry into this specific potential link with peanut allergy.

And so, puzzled doctors moved their attention away from the allergic child to examine the peanut itself. One mystified doctor opined that there "appears to be something unique about the peanut that is not shared by other members of the legume family or most other food proteins."[25]

In analyzing what appeared to make some foods more allergenic than others, researchers focused on three aspects of their proteins: size, abundance, and stability.[26] Proteins are made of strings of amino acids called epitopes. A minimum-size epitope of about thirty amino acids with a molecular weight of 3 kD is required for a protein to cross-link IgE antibodies on the surface of mast cells. If a protein is less than that, it is unable to cross-link IgE, and an allergic response will not result. Peanut proteins (Ara h 1 and Ara h 2) and the soya bean proteins (Gly m 1) have many allergenic epitopes and many IgE binding sites that allow them to cross-link IgE on the surface of mast cells very efficiently. The molecular weight of peanut varies, but Ara h 1 was noted to have a molecular weight of between 20 and 63.5 kDa and Ara h 2 to have a weight of 17kDa.[27]

Peanut proteins are also resistant to degradation by stomach acid and enzymes in the gastrointestinal tract. The "hydrophobic" residues of the amino acids in Ara h 1 peanut epitope, for example, are protected from digestion within the structure of the epitope.[28] They are difficult to digest.

Another "allergenic" feature of proteins is their stability when heated or processed (grinding and cooking). One study claimed that the reason peanut allergy was not seen in China was that people there boil or fry peanuts, which lowers the quantity of Ara h 1 in the peanut (although not its ability to bind to IgE). And compared to dry roasting that was used extensively in the United States, these methods of preparation resulted in a lower level of IgE binding to Ara h 2 and 3. In addition, the high temperature of dry roasting appears to increase the allergenicity of the proteins.[29] According to one researcher, the peanut has adjuvant properties that make it "a perfect allergen."[30]

And consuming a certain protein in a concentrated form may enhance the risk of developing an allergy to it. For example, ovalbumin and ovomucoid that are the two major allergens in chicken egg represent 54% and 11% of the total protein, respectively. Ara h 1 makes up about 16% of the total 24–29% protein of a peanut.[31]

And yet, despite the widely acknowledged allergenicity of peanuts, Americans had been consuming this dietary staple for decades without apparent concern. And given that the allergenicity of peanuts is the same the world over, it could not be used to explain epidemiological features of the allergy—why some countries but not others. Researchers concluded, for example, that the divergent prevalence of the allergy in the United Kingdom compared to Israel "is not accounted for by differences in atopy, social class, genetic background, or peanut allergenicity."[32] Allergenicity, high or low consumption, age of first introduction, all appeared to have little or no bearing on the absence of peanut allergy in Russia and Estonia or its recent emergence in Hong Kong and Singapore in 2007.

A valuable clue existed in the fact of the allergy's sudden increased prevalence in children between 1988 and 1994 in the United Kingdom, the United States, Canada, and Australia. Something in the lives of children changed at that window time that persisted and even worsened through the 2000s—whatever it was, though, the precise role of eating peanuts in the creation of the allergy was far from clear.

TOXIN HYPOTHESIS

First proposed in 1991 by biologist Margie Profet, the toxin hypothesis provided an alternative framework for understanding allergy. It offered, for the first time, a purpose for this disturbing immune response.

IgE is a universal antibody that was programmed millions of years ago. It appears in mammals, marsupials, and nonmammals—including fish and frogs.[33] The evolutionary age of IgE-mediated allergy may be more than sixty million years. Its persistence despite the or because of its damaging effects on the body must have an evolved purpose, argued Profet.

Profet suggested that allergy evolved in mammals as a "last line of defense against toxic substances in the environment in the form of secondary plant compounds and venoms."[34] Because toxins are ubiquitous, humans have developed a variety of tactics to defend against them whether they are inhaled, consumed, rubbed on the skin, or injected (i.e., bee venom). These include the senses of smell and sight, remembering and avoiding, eating a diversity of foods, peeling fruits and vegetables, cooking foods, enzymatic destruction, and shedding epithelial surfaces of organs regularly exposed to toxins, such as in the gut, lungs, and skin.

However, when these primary defenses have previously been unable to stop a specific toxin from entering the bloodstream, allergy is created. The defense tactics of allergy are designed to expel this toxin as quickly as possible from the body.

The chemicals released during an IgE-mediated allergic response can result in vomiting, diarrhea, itching, sneezing, tearing, bronchial constriction, and coughing. These are all ways in which the body is able to expel toxins from the body. The decrease in blood pressure that slows blood flow is an attempt to protect internal organs from potentially circulating toxins.

Profet suggested that nontoxic proteins that become allergens such as peanut are either "reliable correlates" of deemed toxins or carriers of toxins. For example, aflatoxin from mold spores often contaminates peanuts. Allergy to peanuts may actually represent an IgE response to the aflatoxin and, secondarily, to the peanut proteins associated with it.[35] In several allergy studies, mice were made allergic by inhaling or eating peanut mixed with a bacterium—cholera.[36] To create allergy, the body must covalently bind substances (toxin or carrier or both) to serum proteins.

Valency is characterized by the sharing of electrons in a chemical compound—the number of pairs of electrons an atom can share. A valence is an electron ring that encircles the atom. The first ring or valence of any atom can only hold two electrons. The second valence only holds eight. For example, hydrogen has just one valence with one electron and is always looking for a second. Because it is looking to complete its valence, it is reactive and unstable, liable to bind to other elements that are also looking to complete their valence. Oxygen with six electrons in its second valence will bind well to two hydrogen molecules. Together they complete the valence of the other by sharing electrons. Oxygen shares two electrons from the two hydrogen molecules, and each of these shares one from the oxygen molecule. These two elements are covalently bound in a very stable molecule known as water.

Molecules liable to bind more readily with blood serum are those with low molecular weight. Researchers have pointed to the low weight of drugs that must bind to carrier proteins in the body to elicit sensitization (less than 1,000 Da) whereas high molecular weight molecules (larger than 5,000 Da) can act as complete antigens or bind covalently.[37]

The weight of a molecule, measured in Daltons (Da), is the sum of the weights of the atoms (including electrons and protons) of which it is made. For example, the molecular weight of water is 18 Daltons. The molecular weight of the peanut Ara h 1 protein is between 69,000 and 63,500 Daltons or 63.5 kDa. Human IgE antibodies have reacted to three epitopes or strings of amino acids in this protein.[38] Ara h 2 has a molecular weight of 17 kDa. Human IgE identified two binding epitopes in this protein. The *approximate* molecular weights of peanut have been identified: Ara h 3 is about 60 kDa; Ara h 4, 37 kDa; Ara h 5, 15 kDa; Ara h 6, 15 kDa; Ara h 7, 15 kDa; and Ara h 8, 15 kDa.[39]

If the bond between blood serum protein and hapten (a molecule that can elicit an immune response only when bound to the carrier) or carrier is covalent, it is strong and the kidneys cannot filter the hapten. It will continue to circulate in the blood, allowing the immune system to form antibodies to it. A covalent bond between hapten and carrier protein is usually a requirement for the creation of IgE to the hapten.

Proteins that are especially efficient carriers of a wide spectrum of toxic haptens—for example, proteins with hydrophobic pockets that readily bind lipophilic substances, as is the case with the peanut protein—may be the most common targets of IgE antibodies.

But food allergy is not always so linear, Profet reminded readers. It is a complex process by which even two foods consumed together can become linked in the digestive tract if one binds to the toxic hapten of another.[40]

> If allergy is designed to defend against toxins that evade enzymatic detoxification, allergic susceptibility to drugs and ability to detoxify drugs are expected to be inversely related.[41]

In explaining why allergies are more prevalent in industrial societies compared to foraging societies, Profet pointed to exposure over sustained periods to a range of hidden toxins such as food additives or chemicals in soaps and skin creams. These toxins are hard to avoid using general immune defenses. Making matters worse in industrialized society, crowded conditions result in a greater number of respiratory infections that, in turn, are known to increase IgE levels, suggested Profet. This increases allergic sensitivity to the environment.[42]

In contrast, the hygiene hypothesis (below) proposed that the tendency to develop allergies is due to insufficient natural exposure to pathogens rather than an excess exposure. Industrialized societies are protected unnaturally by anti-bacterial products, drugs, and vaccines. In these societies, people are unable to mount a proper immune defense to viral or bacterial pathogens thereby disrupting the Th1/Th2 paradigm. The body favors Th2 that stimulates the production of antibodies including IgE.

At the time of Profet's writing in 1991, the peanut allergy appeared to be just one of a widening range of allergies in Western societies. Since then, no one has picked up the toxin hypothesis and applied it more specifically to the peanut-allergy epidemic in children. Fine-tuning Profet's generalized thesis, perhaps the answer to the specific features of the peanut allergy could have been better understood by unearthing which toxins other than aflatoxin were associated with peanut—whether there were any proteins correlated to or homologous with peanut to which children were being exposed—and which defense systems were failing first or worst when it came to peanut. Precisely how were these associated toxins or correlates with peanut accessing the body?

HELMINTH HYPOTHESIS

Helminths are parasitic worms that live in the human body. It surprised researchers in the 1980s to discover that people heavily infected with certain worms had few allergies. Neil Lynch at the University of Venezuela showed that 90% of Venezuelan Indians living in the rainforest had worms but no allergies. In contrast, when Lynch looked at rich Venezuelans living in the cities, he found that only 10% had light worm infections while 43% had allergies.[43] Similar studies confirmed this feature of certain helminths. An Ethiopian study showed that people infected with hookworm have a low frequency of asthma.[44] A study of helminth-infected Gabonese children showed that a parasite-specific IL10 response in the host suppressed atopy.[45]

From this general "worms versus wealth" concept, researchers developed an explanation for all allergies: because parasites and humans have coevolved, they have a symbiotic relationship in which helminths "protect" humans from developing immune-mediated diseases (colitis, diabetes, etc.) and allergy.[46] According to the theory, while allergy evolved in humans in order to expel helminths, the worms had their own defenses, in turn, that suppressed the human response. However, in the West, hygienic conditions using pesticides and sanitation protocols had largely eliminated helminths from the human population. And without the historic presence of worms, humans were left open to random allergic symptoms.

There are two general categories of helminths: roundworms (ascaris, hookworms, trichinella, filarial, and eye worms); and flatworms (tapeworm, fluke). These worms bury into or latch onto the intestinal wall of their hosts where they feed on blood, cells, and tissue fluids. They lay eggs and reproduce easily. A heavy infection of helminths will lead to their spread from the digestive system into other areas of the body.

But the lack of helminths in the West, again, had left the immune systems of hundreds of thousands of people unbalanced and predictably dysfunctional. Without the suppressing effects of helminths, suggested some researchers, the drive towards the Th2 allergy-inducing side of the immune system is so strong that "bystander proteins" become easy targets for IgE antibodies.[47] The helminth hypothesis explained that without enough parasitic worms in their intestinal tracts, humans are doomed to acquire bowel disease, autoimmune conditions, and allergies.

Identifying this doctor-approved concept as a market opportunity, pharmaceutical companies moved quickly to develop the first worm-based "vaccine" for food allergy.[48] Western doctors also began to offer "worm therapy" to modulate the immune systems of desperate allergy sufferers. The treatment consisted of a deliberate dose of eggs from the pig whipworm, *Trichuris suis* ova (TSO).[49]

But while certain helminth infections can reduce severity of allergic response, additional research indicates that they do not appear to prevent the production of IgE antibodies to any number of allergens. The apparent value of a heavy helminth infection is in making the infected person hyporeactive.[50] For example, where low concentrates of dust mites produced reactions in Dutch subjects, Gabonese children (infected with schistosome) with high IgE to mites needed extremely high concentrations of the allergen before mast cell degranulation was seen.[51]

In fact, extremely high levels of IgE accompany helminth infections. However, much of the IgE was rarely linked to the helminths themselves because, it was suggested, they were efficient at cloaking themselves.[52] Therefore, this mass of IgE was generally believed to be "nonspecific." This mysterious flood of nonspecific antibodies, some researchers offered, prevented mast cell or basophil degranulation by filling up their binding sites. This left little room for additional specific antibodies.[53]

And yet, "if allergy had evolved primarily to protect against helminths, it would represent astonishingly poor design by natural selection."[54] Margie Profet suggested in her research that many of the allegedly "nonspecific" IgE antibodies were actually specific to the excretions and secretions of the helminths that contained toxins absorbed from the host's diet. Helminths produce toxins from which African children with heavy infections have suddenly died.[55]

The helminth hypothesis had other flaws. It could not account for the many phenomena of allergy including why blood pressure drops during a strong allergic response nor why these responses are potentially lethal. Anticoagulants released during allergic reactions appear to have no purpose in defense against helminths. Heparin, however, inhibits the procoagulants of certain snake and insect venoms that fit with the toxin hypothesis. If allergy had evolved to protect against helminths, it made no adaptive sense to Profet.

It seemed unlikely that without worms, humans would malfunction—there were millions of people without heavy worm infections who were equally without Crohn's or ulcerative colitis or allergies. In addition, studies indicated that worms were not the only presence that could suppress allergic reactivity. An infection of *Helicobacter pylori* bacteria was known to dampen allergies. Doctors also suggested that a decreasing prevalence of *H. pylori* in children of industrialized countries might be associated with the epidemics of asthma and allergy.[56] In the end, it seemed more likely that the complete suppression of the immune system by helminths was not symbiotic but rather a straightforward manipulation of the host whose defenses had been neutralized to the advantage of the parasites.

Unchecked, a helminth infection will destroy health and shorten life. The body can produce hydatid cysts containing other cysts and tapeworm heads known as hydatid sand. If a human ingests a hydatid egg, a cyst will develop somewhere in the body. These cysts must be very carefully removed by surgery. If the cyst is punctured and the contents spill into the body, anaphylaxis can occur[57] and each daughter cyst will then mature into additional cysts.

Heavy helminth infections will cause nutritional deficiency, bowel obstruction, appendicitis and peritonitis, anemia, vomiting, internal bleeding, abdominal pain, diarrhea, anorexia, and eosinophilia. The pork tapeworm *Taenia solium* can enter the brain leading to seizures and cysticercosis, as well as parasitic infestation of the central nervous system. For health reasons, some religions have historically forbidden pork consumption.

The host's lymphatic system is also heavily taxed the longer helminths propagate. Their toxic secretions are released into the intestines to be absorbed by the host's bloodstream. This phenomenon makes the host susceptible to viral and bacterial infections.

Ill effects slowly overwhelm a human with a heavy helminth infection. In the meantime, the successful parasite through the fecal matter of the infected person spreads its eggs to other hosts through contaminated water, soil, contact, and food. The spread of worms is enhanced in a society that is poverty stricken, badly nourished, stationary (the people are not foragers), and has lost the knowledge of how to manage parasitic infections through natural means. The inflammation that the helminths suppress is caused by their very presence. Any other benefit conferred through this suppression is coincidental. The purpose of allergy is not to expel helminths and is ineffective at doing so. There was another purpose for the allergic response.

In 2005, researchers suggested that the toxin hypothesis and the helminth hypothesis might fit together in a single causal framework. Allergic reactions intended to kill or expel parasites reduces their toxic effects the most serious of which is bladder cancer. The evolutionary reason for the allergic response may be in minimizing these carcinogenic hazards.[58]

Using the helminth hypothesis to explain the peanut-allergy epidemic, however, was problematic. A study of children in Ghana, Africa, with high levels of IgE to peanut and no clinical reactivity was explained by the suppressing "helminth effect."[59] This same effect, the cornerstone of the theory, does not apply in the United States. Fourteen million Americans ostensibly free of major helminth infections were both sensitized and hyporeactive to peanut. This mass sensitization was identified by an ill-publicized but no less significant US NHANE federal health survey.[60] The survey results of skin prick tests conducted between 1980 and 1994 were not published until 2001. Given the uneven results of skin prick tests, however, one might question that so many were sensitized. But even if half as many were sensitized the point remains. Lack of helminths does not doom one to a life of allergic reactions.

The absence of worms and the idea of a capricious Th2 drive to allergy did not explain the epidemiology of the peanut allergy epidemic. It did not explain why the sudden rise in prevalence of the allergy in western toddlers and why just to peanut (or the other top 7 foods). And given that Western countries have been largely unburdened by major helminth infections for decades, it did not explain the sudden accelerated prevalence of the allergy that began around 1990. Helminths in an investigation of peanut allergy appeared to be coincidental, not causal.

HYGIENE HYPOTHESIS

In 1989, British doctor David Strachan proposed a new explanation for the rise in hay fever, asthma, and allergies. Observing that a decline in family size since the 1960s appeared to correlate with an increase in prevalence of allergy, he speculated on how siblings affect the early development of the immune system. Strachan posited that infection and unhygienic contact with multiple siblings were important lessons for the young immune system. Reduced exposure to viral and bacterial pathogens that would otherwise have been brought home by older siblings and shared with younger ones had led to a skewed system that developed along Th2 rather than Th1 pathways, tending toward allergic conditions.

At the time, doctors were skeptical because most believed that infection was more of a trigger for allergy than a protection. However, the hygiene hypothesis grew in popularity and was supported by the example of Berlin. As already discussed, when the Berlin Wall came down in 1989, curious researchers found that despite the lower levels of hygiene and vaccination and higher levels of pollution and smoking, East Germans rarely suffered from allergy or asthma. Within ten years of reunification, however, allergy affected equal numbers on both sides of the city. Western children, it was then concluded, are too protected from infection by improvements in sanitation, chlorinated water, and medical interventions.[61] Adding to this sheltered existence was the reduced exposure to unhygienic siblings. Thus, the unnatural protections of a Western lifestyle led to a rise in allergy. It seemed to fit.

In a 2000 article, Strachan reiterated his belief in the protective power of infections that were "the most promising candidates" in staving off allergy.[62] The role of vaccination in the development of atopy, however, was dismissed because select studies on measles and pertussis had shown mixed results. And in a 2006 Winnipeg study, it was the two-month delay of vaccination with diphtheria, pertussis, and tetanus (DPT) that was alleged to have allowed children time to develop illness that subsequently cut the prevalence of childhood asthma in half—although there was no evidence that any of the children during those two months had been sick.[63] Researchers insisted that it was not the vaccination that had caused asthma but the alleged natural infections that would have created a balanced and healthy immune system. As well, there seemed limited support for the possible roles of mycobacterial infection and overuse of antibiotics that reduced intestinal flora.

What stood out for Strachan ten years after first proposing the theory were his original findings on variation of hay fever and allergy related to birth order—the tendency to atopy in the first birth and declining in youngest regardless of family size—and socioeconomic status. But these, he suggested, were clues to "the presence of a powerful underlying determinant of allergic sensitization." He suggested that the prevalence of hay fever and asthma was related to one's degree of exposure to this powerful and "true" protective factor.[64] The protective feature of this exposure also appeared to depend on timing.

And so, a renewed hygiene hypothesis in 2000 offered that insufficient exposure to an unknown infectious agent(s) that would afford a robust and balanced Th1/Th2-immune response and therefore protection from allergy was the cause of allergy. Others added the role of regulatory T cell responses (T reg) to this explanation.[65]

But just as the lack of pathogenic stimulation can create allergy, so too can active viral and bacterial diseases acquired naturally or through injection.[66] For example, researchers have correlated the onset of respiratory infections with the onset of IgE-mediated respiratory allergies in children. In one experiment, puppies injected at regular intervals with both pollen extracts and live viral vaccines mounted a significantly greater IgE response than did puppies injected only with pollen extracts.[67] In another example, mice injected with pertussis became allergic to airborne ragweed pollens.[68] The injected pathogens or their toxic die-off acted as adjuvants stimulating the production of IgE.

While children in Ghana who have been exposed to siblings and have many illnesses also have many allergies, these children, however, are hyporeactive; they do not exhibit allergic symptoms to dust mites, for example, because they are "protected" by the immune-suppressing effects of heavy parasitic infections.[69]

The hygiene hypothesis was touted as an explanation not just for asthma and hay fever but also for food allergy. Young, in the *Peanut Allergy Answer Book,* suggested that the absence of infections has "reset" the immune system to target innocuous items in the child's diet resulting in "abnormal" reactions to peanut, for example.

In this explanation without a natural disease burden, the malfunctioning and capricious immune systems of children from too hygienic families have become little more than loose cannons. However, this view could not be reconciled with a basic fact of the peanut allergy epidemic—its sudden acceleration around 1990, in particular.

The hygiene hypothesis does not indicate a functional mechanism of mass sensitization to the peanut. How or why did these proteins or correlates of them access the bloodstreams of these children living in different parts of the Western world at the same time? It had already been established that the role of consumption was mired in confusion in this increased prevalence and that exposure to peanut or cross-sensitizing soy through inhalation or skin cream was equally problematic.

In addtion, the hygiene hypothesis did not offer a purpose for allergy. Given that severe allergy appears in all animals when specific proteins enter and persist in the bloodstream, allergy would have an evolved purpose. As Margie Profet suggested, that purpose is a defense against toxins and any proteins associated with them.

In positing that homeostasis was impossible and allergy virtually assured without a burden of disease, the hygiene hypothesis gave little credit to the human body. Evolutionary biologist Jared Diamond (b. 1937) pointed out that by most accounts, Native Americans had few infectious diseases to give back to the Europeans who landed in the Americas just five hundred years ago.[70] The indigenous hunters and gatherers moved regularly, thus preventing disease that would otherwise occur through the accumulation of toxins and pathogens from animal and human wastes. Conversely, European agricultural-based communities were sedentary. By living in proximity with domestic animals and their wastes, Europeans and other farming societies infected themselves with many viral and bacterial pathogens.

Diamond has suggested that killer diseases are a legacy of ten thousand years of close contact with farm animals. Flu evolved from a disease of pigs transmitted via poultry. Measles was acquired from cattle; and smallpox, some believe, began in camels and moved to cattle. The Incas, unlike the Europeans, did not have the same history of close contact with domesticated animals. The Incas had llamas, but they were not milked, not kept in large herds, and they were not housed next to humans. According to Diamond, there was no significant exchange of germs between llamas and people.

Disease in humans grew from technological and agricultural advances, the consequences of which led to the creation of additional technologies—drugs, vaccines, and antibiotics, which in turn have caused imbalance. In satisfying Strachan's observation that allergic sensitization was related to the timing and intensity of human exposure to a powerful underlying determinant, perhaps technology and its concomitant toxicities begged a closer look.

EXPANDED HYGIENE HYPOTHESIS

The original hygiene hypothesis proposed by Strachan in 1989 suggested that without adequate exposure to specific pathogens humans are virtually doomed to allergy. The protections of sanitation and limited germ exposure had unhinged the immune systems of infants. Surprisingly, antibiotics and vaccination seemed to play no role in the theory. By 2014, however, researchers had begun to look at the obvious and study the destructive nature of antibiotics on gut ecology.

In 2014, a study from the University of Chicago Medical Center indicated that clostridia, strains of this common gut bacterium, helped reduce allergic sensitization. In the study, mice were treated with antibiotics which destroyed the clostridia then force-fed peanut. Blood samples from the mice then indicated an increase in IgE, the 'allergy antibody.' However, when clostridia was re-introduced to their digestive tracts the mice experienced a reduction antibody production specific to the peanut.

According to study authors, "Clostridia caused innate immune cells to produce high levels of interleukin-22 (IL-22), a signaling molecule known to decrease the permeability of the intestinal lining."[71]

Of great importance, as discussed in Chapter 2: Risk Factors, is that while sensitized to peanut none of the mice actually reacted to the food.

In contrast, a 2013 study glossed over clostridia but identified bacteroides fragilis as important in food tolerance but only if introduced in the neonatal period. Clearly, much research needed to be done on the cultivation of these gut 'bugs' and their role in the enteric immune system.

Children receive an average of 2.2 antibiotic prescriptions in the first year of life according to a 2013 study. The study looked at two groups of children born between 2007 and 2009—those diagnosed with food allergies and those without. In this study, children who had had 2.65 antibiotic exposures compared to 1.84 exposures were at greater risk for food allergies as measured by IgE antibodies. The study speculated on the destructive impact antibiotics have on digestive flora and how this contributes to sensitization.[72]

Again, as reviewed in chapter 2, children are commonly prescribed antibiotics for ear and throat bacterial infections, often from strep.

Between 1988 and 1994, there was a significant increase in ear infections among US children.[73] In this time frame, the number of children with ear infections under one year of age went up by 3% and recurrent ear infections (3 or more) increased by 6%—this latter figure representing an increase of 720,000 more children in the 6 year period.

An important question at this point in the 'expanded hygiene hypothesis' is to ask what was causing this soaring increase in ear infections for which antibiotics were prescribed? Many doctors and naturopaths point to back undiagnosed food allergies especially to dairy.

In a 1994 *Annals of Allergy* study, 86% of children had a significant reduction in ear infections simply by eliminating allergenic foods from their diet (wheat, eggs, corn, etc.).[74]

Dairy allergy often goes undiagnosed although its causal role in ear infections has been known for decades.

ENT specialist Dr. David Hurst has dedicated a web site to the role of allergy in ear infections stating that "allergy is the cause of most chronic middle ear fluid, and that aggressive use of standardized allergy management can solve the problem":

> It is my contention that the middle ear behaves like the rest of the respiratory tract and that what has been learned about the allergic response in the sinuses and lungs may be applied to the study of the ear to help in understanding the pathophysiology of chronic otitis media with effusion (OME).[75]

Again, if the root cause of ear infection is allergy that in turn causes inflammation and invites infection for which antibiotics are required, *what caused the initial allergies?*

This appears to be a circular discussion. However, one might suspect that while antibiotics make one more vulnerable to sensitization there is yet another sensitizing mechanism at play such as vaccination which is a well known and immediate cause of allergy and anaphylaxis.

With vaccination the goal of immunity and allergy are inseparable—both defenses are provoked simultaneously. Although a known method of sensitization for well over 100 years, vaccination remained out of bounds for any researcher keen on keeping his or her job. And yet, the role of vaccines seems to fit easily into the expanded hygiene hypothesis. NY allergist Dr. Scott Sicherer stated in an email to Fox News in 2012 (available online):

> The leading theory is about hygiene-with less infection thanks to city living, smaller families, vaccines, sanitation, antibiotics, etc. . . .[76]

While the hygiene hypothesis had expanded to include pharmaceuticals, it could not as yet include vaccination.

Part 2

A HISTORY OF MASS ALLERGY

Chapter 4

—∞∞∞—

REDISCOVERING ANAPHYLAXIS

At the close of the 19th century there emerged suddenly a peculiar child-specific illness so widespread that new words had to be created to describe it: allergy and anaphylaxis. The illness characterized by hives, inflammation, vomiting, shock and drop in blood pressure was a side effect of a technology and procedure never before used together in mass application—vaccination with the hypodermic syringe.

Although asthma and eczema were common if minor concerns prior to the 1890s, documented life-threatening and anaphylactic-like reactions were few and indeed the reaction itself appears to have been relatively rare in history. A story of anaphylaxis was told in hieroglyphs regarding the reaction of Pharaoh Menes who died in 2640 BC from a wasp sting.[1] Hippocrates (460–375) described reactions to foods such as dairy that roused "a constituent of the body which is hostile to cheese." A fatality to a sting was reported by a French physician in 1765, thought to be the first documented case in Europe.

In the nineteenth century, French physiologist François Magendie (1783–1855) found that animals sensitized to egg white by injection went into shock and died after a subsequent injection.[2] Similar violent reactions in humans were believed to be rare "idiosyncrasies" that London doctor Jonathan Hutchinson (1828–1913) called individuality run mad.[3] At the close of the nineteenth century and the start of the twentieth, however, such reactions began to appear with startling frequency particularly in children. These reactions were produced following the application of a new technology, the hypodermic syringe to administer antitoxin sera in the revolutionary treatment called vaccination.

Public tolerance of vaccination-induced anaphylaxis and allergy, then simply called serum sickness, was weighed against the fear of acquiring diseases in their natural form. Serum sickness with which vaccine makers and doctors struggled for decades into the 20th century was not understood until after 1901. At the dawn of the twentieth century, immunologist and Nobel laureate Charles Richet and pediatrician Clemens von Pirquet were able to show how the injection had caused the first allergy epidemic in children.

JUSTIFIED BEHAVIOR IN THE FIRST LANCET VACCINATION

Vaccination was developed in response to rampant and deadly infectious diseases in the Western world. Many of these diseases in European and Asian societies had become a problem centuries ago when wastes from animal husbandry—the domestication of animals like cow, goat, pig, chicken, and sheep—transferred viral and bacterial pathogens to humans. Unlike the hunter-gatherer societies, farming societies offered a more sedentary lifestyle in which just a few farmers could produce enough food for many people. Towns and villages grew up around the farms that flourished using plows, irrigation, and manure fertilization. However, the inevitable runoff of human and animal fecal matter with accompanying intestinal parasites and other contaminants drained into streams and rivers, infecting local sources of drinking water.

Again, as Jared Diamond pointed out, the Native American hunting and gathering societies had few diseases to give back to the Europeans when they arrived in the New World.[4] Many indigenous populations like the Aztec and Incas in South America and the Huron and other tribes in North America were decimated by European smallpox and other deadly illnesses.

And arguably no less were Europeans devastated by their own diseases. Enhanced agricultural technologies in Europe meant that fewer people were required to work on farms. Without livelihood, uprooted populations crowded into larger industrialized communities looking for work. Densely populated cities like London or Paris that lacked proper waste disposal protocols until the mid to late nineteenth century encouraged the spread of disease—whether bubonic plague from the bite of infected fleas carried by rats or cholera from water contaminated with human feces.

These migrant peoples lured by the promise of land in North America also crowded onto ships. En route to their destinations, illness often swept through the close confines shared by hundreds of travelers. Once landed, health officials examined all arrivals, and those who appeared ill were imprisoned in large quarantine tents. Use of pestilence or "pest" houses was also a common method of segregating the sick and attempting to contain contagious diseases.

Faced with a flood of immigrants and the threat of epidemic disease, officials required new laws and protocols for managing the waste and other problems that grew from crowding thousands of people into one small geographical area—London was the largest city in the world in 1900 with a population of about one million. This urbanizing trend, also called the social problem, forced many cities to formally incorporate and to develop departments of health to deal with bacteriology and disinfection.

Thus, the unnatural conditions of Western progress—the shift from hunter-gatherer to agrarian and thence to industrial-based societies—necessitated all manner of technical innovations not the least of which were in disease management. Fundamental to maintaining the health of Westernized city populations were the sanitation of water systems, methods of waste disposal, and the development of medicines and vaccines—which in turn seemed to produce new problems such as adverse reactions like allergy and anaphylaxis. Agriculture, Diamond reiterated, "was in many ways the greatest catastrophe from which we have never recovered."[5]

In the eighteenth century, smallpox, also known as variola, was a common and deadly disease that was often treated with infrequent success by variolation or inoculation. This technique named from the Latin word *inoculare* (to graft) referred to the use of a lancet or sharp pronged tool used to remove matter from a pustule of a smallpox victim and then to apply it under the skin—on the arm or leg—of a nonimmune person. Any risk assumed from this crude treatment may have seemed more than justified when compared to acquiring the disease naturally at the time. There was an estimated 20% to 60% chance of death from the terrifying natural form of smallpox acquired by two-thirds of the population of Western Europe in the mid-eighteenth century. Well-justified fear easily dominated the conscious mind that was witness to so many agonizing deaths.

The worst strain of smallpox was black pox. Black pox caused the eyes to become dark red pits and the skin darkened with hemorrhaging blood, to "slip off the body in sheets."[6] Ordinary smallpox caused the entire body, inside and out, to bubble up in painful infected blisters. When these pustules lost their pressure, they leaked liters of the odorous pus until they finally crusted over in brown scabs. But the scabbing phase could be the most dangerous. Just as a victim seemed to have improved, it was common for the patient to suddenly bleed out internally oozing liquid from every orifice. Smallpox left the brain for last. Victims remained fully aware of their condition with their appetites intact until the end. Those who survived the disease were hideously scarred. And one-third of these were left blind.[7]

Vaccination was initially developed to combat smallpox. When an outbreak occurred in Gloucestershire, England, in 1788, country doctor Edward Jenner (1749–1823) observed that people, such as dairymaids, who worked with cattle, had much milder cases of the disease. As the legend is often told, Jenner deduced a connection between cowpox and smallpox and began to experiment with cow pus variolation. One of his first experiment volunteers was an eight-year-old boy. Jenner made wounds on the boy's skin and applied a liquid made from cowpox sores. After the patient's recovery from the milder cowpox, Jenner applied a smallpox liquid in the same manner. When the patient did not contract the disease, Jenner was able to repeat his experiment on several children and adults. This time he used an arm-to-arm "passive" treatment, transferring pus from one person to another. Only four of these people were challenged by smallpox and found to be protected.

Jenner was subsequently lionized by the medical community as a hero whose experiments on children laid the foundation for disease management through childhood vaccination. Jenner's technique that he called vaccination in 1798 after the Latin word *vacca* for *cow* did have a precedent in at least one documented case in England. Farmer Benjamin Jesty (1737–1816) in the 1770s inoculated his own family using a darning needle and cow pus.

At his own expense, Jenner published his results—twelve experiments plus sixteen additional case histories he had collected since the 1770s—in the *Inquiry into the Causes and Effects of the Variolae Vaccine* (1798). This text was translated into a variety of languages—including French, Italian, and Dutch—thereby introducing the vaccination technique to many countries.[8]

Jenner's work and the hope it engendered resulted in mass vaccination campaigns throughout Europe. By 1821, Denmark, Norway, Russia, Sweden, and others had made infant vaccination compulsory. Vaccination was even taken to the Caribbean. In 1803, King Charles IV of Spain sent Francisco Xavier de Balmis to their colonies in the Americas on the Royal Philanthropic Expedition of the Vaccine. Before leaving Spain, De Balmis kidnapped five Madrid orphans for the voyage. During the voyage, one child after the other was made ill with cowpox through arm-to-arm vaccination. In this way De Balmis kept the vaccine fresh until they arrived at their destination.[9]

Reflecting on the ethics of Jenner's experiments on children, one modern researcher stated that the doctor was justified given the devastating nature of smallpox at that time.[10] Jenner gambled his own life as well in this medical venture. The death of a child might have led to a charge of murder. And yet, patients embraced the cards of risk and reward dealt by the procedure. It was the lesser of two evils, and if there were side effects, the patient gratefully assumed all responsibility for them.

It was soon discovered, however, that a single vaccination did not confer lifelong immunity. As well, inconsistent vaccination procedures used by doctors had actually led to the spread of cowpox and other diseases. Creative doctors would scratch or puncture the skin using a variety of unsanitary tools such as knives, forks, needles and pins in parallel, crosshatch, spiral, and geometric formations.[11] And the passive arm-to-arm vaccination method frequently transmitted secondary infections, including leprosy and syphilis. Syphilis, called the great pox, was terrifying and fatal. Infections or "poisons" introduced by lancet wounds could also result in the loss of use of the vaccinated arm or in its ultimate amputation.[12]

Under these conditions, the challenge of safe vaccine delivery seemed insuperable. A vaccine had to be created, transported, and then administered. And it had to be done as safely as possible. Initially, an infected calf provided a fresh source of cowpox vaccine. The animal was led by foot or shipped from town to town where doctors or others would use the pus in the tradition of Jenner. Eventually, however, the calf would either recover or die thus ending the supply. In desperate times, cowpox scabs were packaged and mailed and then reconstituted. Finally, an antibacterial vegetable glycerin was added to liquid cowpox pus.[13] This mixture naturally decomposed within a short period, prompting vaccine makers to include preservatives.

Despite the inconsistent results of Jenner's technology, it opened up the potential for managing other diseases in the same manner. The rapid speed with which vaccination and indeed technology of all kinds evolved during the nineteenth century was marked by impatience on the part of scientists.

Scientists Theodor Schwann and Mathias Schleiden in 1839 published the idea that plants and animals were made of cells, from the Latin *cellular* or *room*. It was a short step from cell biology to germ theory, a concept that marked the beginning of modern science-based medicine. Louis Pasteur (1822–1895) refuted the idea that disease was spontaneously generated from ghostlike miasms. Disease was a manifestation of microorganisms in the environment or in the body. His German rival Koch used a microscope to identify in 1882 and 1883 respectively, the germs that caused tuberculosis and cholera.

And yet, the idea that invisible germs could make one sick was an astonishing idea. Even doctors had a hard time accepting the concept when it was first posited in a clinical setting. Hungarian physician Dr. Ignaz Semmelweis (1818–1865) in 1847 outraged his contemporaries by suggesting that just by washing their hands, doctors could save thousands of women from death in childbirth. Imprudently, Semmelweis persisted vociferously in his beliefs until his frightened wife believed he was losing his mind. In 1865, she had him committed to an asylum where he died two weeks later allegedly beaten to death by guards.

The public, too, resisted the idea that invisible germs were in the air, food, and water. In 1854, renowned public health worker John Snow had to convince London officials that an outbreak of cholera in Soho was being caused by a particular communal water well contaminated by human feces. Snow pioneered shoe-leather epidemiology, going door-to-door to trace the source of the outbreak. Finally, city officials removed the pump handle from a well on Broad Street thus ending the outbreak.

Such public breakthroughs gave doctors and men of science a new gloss of authority and social prestige—even the word *scientist* was new having just been coined in 1833 by English polymath William Whewell (1794–1866). Through the nineteenth century, there emerged a parade of scientific innovations that produced both exciting and destabilizing effects. None of the technological advances was without problem or further opportunity.

An electric distribution system patented in 1880 by Thomas Edison allowed him to capitalize on his invention of the electric lamp (one of his 1,093 US patents), spawning an explosion in electric devices. Scottish-born Alexander Graham Bell (1847–1922) patented the telephone in 1876 and engendered a communications revolution. German inventor and engineer Karl Benz (1844–1929) patented an internal combustion engine in 1879 for use in automobiles; he built the first horseless carriage, the patented Motorwagen in 1885. The appeal of the automobile spurred the evolution of a massive petroleum industry (begun in 1846 with a method of refining it into kerosene).

Other nineteenth-century inventions that had significance in daily life included the typewriter and the qwerty keyboard, the sewing machine, the toaster, the tin can (and the can opener), and, the invention that marked the entire century, mass production of all of these new devices.

Having no less an impact during this period of rapid industrialization and modernization was the rise of mass vaccination that grew from the success of Jenner and a long line of heroes in the study of immunology. On the heels of Jenner, Pasteur, and Koch, scientists from France, Germany, and England raced to develop vaccines—these countries funded and encouraged scientific advance because it enhanced their international profiles and because it led to improved technologies of war such as biological and chemical warfare. These two goals seemed to come together in 1896 when the estate of Swedish inventor Alfred Nobel (1833–1896) revealed the multimillionaire's will had established a fund with five prizes, three of which were for science.

Nobel who had made a fortune from his patented nitroglycerin dynamite was startled by the publication in 1888 of a premature obituary which called him a "merchant of death": "Dr. Alfred Nobel, who became rich by finding ways to kill more people faster than ever before, died yesterday." From this, allegedly, Nobel was moved to create the $9-million fund for the prizes as a more positive lasting legacy—especially in science.

The news of the Nobel prizes intensified the already-heated competition between international vaccine scientists. In the first decade of the prizes, the majority of prizes in medicine went to those working on disease: the first Nobel Prize in Physiology and Medicine in 1901 went to Emil von Behring "for his work in serum therapy against diphtheria"; the 1902 prize went to Ronald Ross (United Kingdom, 1857–1932) "for his work on malaria"; in 1903 it was Niels Ryberg Finsen (Denmark, 1860–1904) for his work on lupus vulgaris and other diseases; 1905 to Robert Koch (Germany, 1843–1910) for his work in tuberculosis; 1907 to Charles Laveran (France, 1845–1922) for his understanding of protozoa in causing diseases; 1908 to Ilya Illyich Mechnikov (Russia, 1845–1916) and Paul Ehrlich (Germany, 1854–1915) for "their work on immunity."

Ingredients for a variety of vaccines evolved rapidly through the late nineteenth and early twentieth centuries in order to extend vaccine shelf life to make them more effective and to reduce prevalence of adverse events including serum sickness that simply could not be eliminated. Such ingredients eventually included a mercury-based antifungal, oil excipients to enhance the reactivity of the body, carrier gels made from boiled animals, and more. Exact ingredients of these proprietary formulae held by commercial vaccine makers—and benefiting the scientists who developed them—were fiercely guarded by patent and corporate law, the cornerstone of which was shareholder protection. These protections and new legislation to help protect the public from vaccine damage grew within an economic framework supported by the tradition of mass vaccination.

A FRAMEWORK FOR MASS VACCINATION

Research and development in vaccines was aided by the invention of a new device making their administration easier and more effective, the hypodermic needle. At the same time, laying the framework for the production, distribution, and sale of both vaccine and needle were the business-minded makers of patent medicines and pharmaceuticals. These proliferated in large numbers at the close of the US Civil War (1861–65).

The Civil War created an unprecedented demand for pharmaceuticals (from the Greek *pharmakon* or *remedy*), including painkillers, anesthetics, and smallpox vaccination materials. More soldiers on both Union and Confederate sides succumbed to disease than were killed in action. While an estimated three hundred thousand Union soldiers died during the war, only one-third of these deaths were from war wounds. In deciding the outcome of the war, smallpox was a significant factor whether acquired naturally or deliberately through its use as a bioweapon. There was at least one documented example of a Confederate doctor who knowingly sold smallpox-infected clothes to Union soldiers.[14]

Soldiers were expected to be vaccinated using the lancet, and they welcomed it. The vaccine medium consisted of glycerin and pulverized crusts or scabs from cowpox pustules obtained from vaccinated calves or children. However, late in the war, there was a shortage of all medicines, including scabs. These, naturally, became valuable. Private physicians were paid $5 (about $70 in 2008) for each usable scab.[15] Some soldiers collected scabs and sent them home for their families to use and possibly sell. With drug shortages, blockade running or smuggling were methods by which doctors hoped to obtain these scabs and other drugs, including quinine, chloroform, ether, opium, and morphine. In lieu of these, desperate doctors and druggists resorted to old remedy recipes using barks, leaves, and roots of native plants. They used butterfly root for fever, red-oak bark and bicarbonate of soda as antiseptics, and poppy heads and nightshade to reduce pain.

Wartime lessons in creative drug innovation and the cost-effective mass manufacture of the same had made business in pharmaceuticals potentially profitable. Aided by aggressive marketing and the expansion in the medicines industry north of the Mason-Dixon Line demand for cures of all kinds grew.

Many small companies sprang up at the close of the Civil War. Companies such as Upjohn (established in Michigan, 1885) made heart pills with nitroglycerin, digitalis, strophanthus, and belladonna. Eli Lilly and Company, launched in 1876 by Civil War veteran and pharmacist Eli Lilly, produced cannabis tinctures, poisons, gelatin capsules for liquid medicines, and succus alternas, a blood purifier for syphilis derived from a Creek Indian remedy.[16]

The late nineteenth-century makers and sellers of patent or trademarked medicines on both sides of the Atlantic were dubbed "nostrum-mongers" by novelist Henry James—their products or *nostrum remedium* ("our remedy") in Latin was shortened to *nostrum*.

Patented nostrums that grew from 2,700 in 1880 to 38,000 by 1916 tended to have high alcohol content and were fortified with morphine, opium, or cocaine. Late nineteenth-century remedies such as the German imported Bayer's powdered heroin hydrochloride intended to cure morphine addiction, Lloyd Brothers Cannabis in alcohol for gonorrhea, John Wyeth & Bros. morphine and chloroform cough syrup, or Mulford Co.'s cotton-root bark abortion tincture were doubtlessly dangerous. These nostrums were sold using aggressive media campaigns that included print advertising, trademarks, lively packaging, and promotional vehicles such as medical almanacs. The companies used saturation advertising and employed newspaper agents in the distribution of mail-order products.[17]

Nostrum mongers frequently exaggerated the curative power of their remedies. Henry James's psychologist brother, William James, was so appalled by "the medical advertisement abomination" that in 1894 he declared that "the authors of these advertisements should be treated as public enemies and have no mercy shown."[18] And yet, many of these nostrum sellers in continuing to embrace advances in Western medicine and science grew into profitable modern pharmaceutical companies.

Parke-Davis (est. 1866, Detroit) that began in the sale of herbal remedies became the largest US pharmaceutical company with annual sales of more than $3 million in the 1890s—the rough equivalent in 2008 of $73 million. This company dominated the vaccine market that grew quickly beyond just smallpox. Next to "modified mixed infection" vaccines—with license No. 1 issued in 1902 by the Secretary of the Treasury USA—the company sold such remedies as cocaine tablets to cure morphine addiction and buttermilk pills for invalids.

In the nostrum-monger tradition, Parke-Davis founded medical publications such as the influential *Therapeutic Gazette* (published by company co-owner George S. Davis)[19] and supported others such as the *Index Medicus*, an index guide to medical journal articles catalogued initially by US Army doctor and booklover John Shaw Billings (1838–1913). Parke-Davis also collaborated with members of the academic medical community, recruiting some for its research labs as it did in 1895 when it hired E. M. Houghton from the University of Michigan. By the 1890s, companies were able to hire workers trained in bacteriology, which was for the first time offered in medical school curricula.

As the US economy expanded, pharmaceutical companies enlarged both their manufacturing operations and their sales forces so that they were able to reach the doctors who were servicing fast-growing urban populations across the country.

The marketing methods for vaccines and antitoxins in the 1890s resembled those used for pharmaceuticals today. Pharma company sales reps visited physicians to market the products and left promotional sales literature, including reprints of medical articles. One pamphlet quoted diphtheria fatality rates of 34.8% to 62.5% without antitoxin, but 4.6% to 17.6% with it.[20] Parke-Davis competitor Mulford Co. was aggressive in its sales literature for diphtheria antitoxin telling doctors, "Don't be afraid to use the antitoxin. Don't be afraid of a large dose. Don't wait for result of a culture before use." Similarly, an 1897 Parke-Davis advertisement proclaimed, "We have never yet had reported a case of sudden death following the use of our antitoxin."[21] However, by 1901–1902 there were several deaths related to the commercially produced smallpox and diphtheria vaccines.

Diphtheria, dubbed the "strangling angel," is a bacterial infection that causes the lymph glands, throat, and neck to swell. In severe cases, the patient can suffocate. A milder form of diphtheria can also create skin lesions. Between

1891–1900 in London, there were 2.98 deaths from diphtheria per 1,000 children under age five; between 1891–94 there were 548 deaths in the city. This rate was lower outside the major cities.[22]

In the 1890s, the German physician Emil von Behring developed an "antitoxic" or protective serum that did not kill the diphtheria bacterium, but rather helped neutralize the toxic poisons that the bacterium released into the body. Von Behring created the antitoxin from the blood (serum) of patients infected with diphtheria and from vaccinated animals. Von Behring first successfully used his antitoxin serum on a child with the disease in 1891. His vaccine was likely the single most important catalyst in the creation of the science-based pharmaceutical industry.[23] It brought him considerable wealth and fame.

Mass production and administration of the antitoxin sera followed this success. Commercial and government laboratories used blood from farm animals in order to meet the enormous demand for the vaccine.[24] Horses were thought ideal animals in which to produce antitoxin because they were large and highly reactive to diphtheria. A report in *The New York Times* told the story of one horse worth $175,000 to the City of New York.[25] Used by the Street Cleaning Department, horse 397 was ready for the glue factory when an enterprising doctor recruited him for the New York Health Department's Otisville laboratories (established in 1894). The horse was infected with diphtheria and bled twice a week, producing 232,800,000 units of antitoxin over two years.

The mass vaccination of children with such antitoxin sera resulted in an apparent reduction in mortality rates. More than thirty articles heralded this outcome in the popular press in the United States in 1894 and 1895. Despite the success, however, injections were well known to cause a poorly understood and potentially fatal illness known at this time as "serum sickness."

Lab animals and horses repeatedly immunized with tetanus or diphtheria antigens to produce the antisera were often afflicted with serum sickness. Horses were known to suddenly collapse and die after a second or third injection. In humans, the condition made headlines after the daughter of renowned pathologist Paul Langerhans died within minutes of a diphtheria antiserum injection. In fact, serum sickness ravaged thousands of children causing fevers, rash, diarrhea, falling blood pressure, joint pain, breathing difficulties, and other symptoms.

Diphtheria serum deaths soon made headlines in Norway, Hungary, in 1895 and in the United States in 1901.[26] In 1901, a five-year-old child was admitted to a St. Louis hospital for treatment of a diphtheria infection. She received two antitoxin shots. Nine days later, she died from tetanus. An ensuing investigation revealed that the Health Department for the City of St. Louis had produced diphtheria antitoxin using a horse that had died of tetanus—the horse had been used to produce in excess of thirty quarts of antitoxin over a three-year period. Two flasks of serum from the deceased horse were reportedly dumped down a laboratory sink. In reality, it was shown that the batch had actually been distributed to physicians. An additional twelve children died from tetanus shortly after the first. Another one hundred cases of postvaccinal tetanus occurred in New Jersey in 1901 with nine fatalities. The media called these children antitoxin victims.[27]

A standard for diphtheria antitoxin had been developed in 1895 by the Hygienic Laboratory, an arm of the US Marine Hospital Service. The lab was later renamed the Public Health Service. While the government produced vaccines alongside corporate enterprises at this time, the Hygienic Laboratory officials warned of "what will evidently ensue in our country. Many persons will commence to prepare the (anti-diphtheria) serum as a business enterprise, and there will, without a doubt, be many worthless articles called antitoxin thrown upon the market. All the serum intended for sale should be made or tested by competent persons."[28]

Government's role in building the tradition of vaccination gradually shifted from production to purely regulatory and administrative. Regulatory intervention began with the 1902 Biologics Control Act, making the Hygienic Laboratory responsible for issuing licenses to makers of biologics that included vaccines—thirteen businesses were licensed in 1904. This number grew quickly from twenty-four businesses in 1908 to forty-one in 1921 producing over one hundred biologics.[29]

But safety was not the only vaccine related concern of government. In 1906, a charge of conspiracy in price fixing was brought against the Drug Trust of the United States. The Proprietary Association (for holders of patent medicines) and the Wholesale and Retail Druggists Associations as well as certain individuals were charged with violating Sherman Antitrust laws.[30] In addition, there were long-held concerns regarding false and misleading nostrum advertising that reporter Samuel Adams (1871–1958) called the Great American Fraud in Collier's Weekly (1905). The Pure Food and Drug Act passed in 1906 attempted to control false claims related to ingredients. These government actions helped restore public confidence in vaccination.

Despite the apparent acrimonious relationship—the lawsuits and tightening controls that continued with a 1936 ban on the use of certain ingredients such as alcohol and narcotics—government needed pharmaceutical companies and their vaccines. Vaccination, its easy administration and promise of better odds against disease, was logically tied to the government's bottom line, economic growth. A sick population spelled the financial decline of a city or even a country. And they knew from bitter lessons learned during the US Civil War that a disease-afflicted army could lose.

The tradition of compulsory injections for US soldiers began in World War I (1914–1918) with vaccines for typhoid, cholera, tetanus, smallpox, and other diseases. For the nostrum-mongers that had grown into lucrative science-based pharmaceutical companies, the government was a valuable customer that could and would influence and even enforce the buying decisions of the public. This seesaw relationship was woven into a complex fabric of conflicting concerns and desires that included the reputations and incomes of doctors and scientists and the interests of powerful medical associations, shareholders, the authority of government, and the media—which in its turn was supported by rich ad sales from pharmaceutical companies. The net result was a pattern of increasing drug and vaccine consumption in Western industrialized countries that transformed the patient into a medical consumer.[31]

THE NEGLECTED ROLE OF THE NEEDLE: DISCOVERING THE TWIN RELATIONSHIP OF IMMUNITY & ALLERGY

Medical consumers gradually embraced the tradition of vaccination by injection. Any concerns they had about the treatment focused naturally on reactions to the vaccine ingredients—the "antitoxin" victims a case in point. In the creation of these poorly understood adverse reactions, however, few seemed aware of the significant role and meaning of the device that had made modern vaccination possible, the hypodermic needle.

The syringe with a needle fine enough to pierce the skin was developed independently in 1853 by Frenchman physician Charles Pravaz (1791–1853) and Scottish physician Alexander Wood (1817–1884). It was Wood, however, who in 1858 first publicized his "hypodermic" or beneath-the-skin needle as an ideal method for introducing morphine directly into the bloodstream. Wood's paper "A New Method of Treating Neuralgia by the Direct Application of

Opiates to the Painful Points" in the *Edinburgh Medical and Surgical Review* reported excellent results. The needle, which made the effect of morphine, a principal ingredient of opium,[32] at once immediate and more powerful than ingestion, was rapidly embraced by doctors and by the public in Europe and America. Florence Nightingale (1820–1910), pioneering nurse of the Crimean War (1853–56), wrote during her later years of illness, "Nothing did me any good, but a curious little new fangled operation of putting opium under the skin which relieved one for twenty-four hours."

The convenience and enhanced potency offered by this direct introduction to the bloodstream contributed to the increased prevalence of opiate addiction. Injected morphine used by doctors to treat the wounded during the US Civil War resulted in an alleged postwar malady called soldier's disease—in effect, thousands of veterans were made addicts. While this assertion has been debated, it remains a fact that the needle led to a rise in the medical and nonmedical demand for morphine and its derivatives. One derivative was heroin, which was brought to market by Bayer in 1898. Morphine addiction was also the ultimate outcome for the hypodermic inventor Wood as well as his wife. Her eventual overdose is believed to have been the first such recorded death.

The first doctor to use the hypodermic needle to inject a vaccine was Louis Pasteur. His initial use of the device in the development of his anthrax vaccine for livestock[33] was followed in 1885 by vaccination of a young boy who had been bitten by a rabid dog.[34] Until Pasteur, vaccination referred only to cowpox and smallpox. Pasteur redefined vaccine as live or inactivated microorganisms (bacteria, viruses) injected in order to induce immunity and to help prevent infectious disease.

Gradually, the hypodermic needle began to replace the unsteady and messy transdermal tools that were used to puncture or scratch the skin. There were few obstacles to the widespread use of the needle for vaccination. The cost was reasonable at $2.50 per device in 1897 (about $67 in 2008). Improvements on the design were required—the glass barrels tended to crack, tips leaked, and needles easily snapped.

Production of liquid vaccines suited to the features of the hypodermic needle quickly followed. Vaccines in vegetable glycerin were developed for scarlet fever, yellow fever, snakebite, tuberculosis, and more by the end of the century. Vaccines were mass produced, packaged in vials, and then stored and shipped to doctors in distant places. The needle made the mass administration of vaccines convenient, cost effective, and relatively sanitary; the reuseable metal needles could be boiled or dipped in alcohol to kill bacteria. The graduated scale on the side of the glass barrel meant that serum could be measured. This was especially important given the noticeably stronger and immediate effects of injection.

Oral administration of drugs reduced and slowed their effects because of the natural action of digestive enzymes that destroyed and eliminated them. Injection seemed to be a better method of administration because it made the drug more potent. In the application of vaccines, however, bypassing the protections of digestion and skin to inject deep into body tissues would prove to be far more problematic.

The convenient packaging of the needle with antitoxin starting in the 1890s had wholly unforeseen outcomes. The shot pried the lid off a Pandora's box and unwittingly exposed those vaccinated to a host of manmade chronic degenerative diseases. The first was the life-threatening allergic condition known as serum sickness. Doctors struggled to prevent serum sickness, "the great bane of serum therapy" as it was called in a 1919 paper on the subject. [J.H. Lewis, "Slow intravenous injection of antiserum to prevent acute anaphylactic shock," JAMA, Vol. 72, No. 5 (Feb. 1919): p. 329.] While vaccine innovation gradually reduced although never eliminated the prevalence of serum sickness as the century unfolded (horses and sheep as sources for antitoxin were replaced by lab samples such as chicken embryos and small animals), this episode in the history of vaccination provided an open window onto the ease with which allergic conditions can be created by the expedient of injection.

SERUM SICKNESS: A PRECEDENT FOR AN ALLERGY EPIDEMIC IN CHILDREN

Serum sickness was a condition that included the then yet-to-be-named allergy and anaphylaxis. The sickness in children was a common outcome of the first mass injections of antitoxin sera for scarlet fever, tetanus, and diphtheria before the turn of the century. Symptoms of serum sickness ranged from rashes, joint pain, fever, lymph node swelling, decreased blood pressure, enlarged spleen, kidney failure, breathing difficulty, and shock, which sometimes killed the patient.[35]

With the mass administration of injected sera, sickness occurred according to one writer in 1941 about "once in every seven hundred treatments" in the early decades of the twentieth century.[36] Another writer put that number much higher with a 10% chance of developing acute serum sickness.[37] Yet another in 1934 believed it to be 50% of vaccinated children.[38] The immediate effects of postvaccinal serum sickness could last days, weeks, months, or might never clear, leaving the victim in a chronic state of ill health and reactive to a range of substances including the vaccines themselves.

Austrian pediatrician Clemens Von Pirquet (1874–1929) and his Hungarian colleague Béla Schick (1877–1967) studied serum sickness in thousands of children subjected to injections of antitoxic sera. In his detailed examinations of the children at the Universitats Kinderklinik in Vienna, Von Pirquet showed that the diverse manifestations of serum sickness were similar to those noted in hypersensitive reactions to strawberries, crabs, pollens, and the poisons of bees and mosquitoes.

Von Pirquet postulated a close and seemingly paradoxical relationship between the two outcomes of vaccination: the process of becoming immunized and the hypersensitive characteristics of serum sickness. In both cases, there was an incubation period between initial injection and appearance of symptoms; subsequent injections (like secondary exposure to infection) were accompanied by accelerated and exaggerated responses resulting from "a collision of antigen and antibody."[39]

There were, he also noted, idiosyncrasies or individual variations in response to sera related to dose and injection intervals. Immediate adverse reaction in 90% of his patients had occurred following the second injections ten to thirty days after the first. Von Pirquet concluded that the length of incubation time depended not only upon the foreign body or antigen but also upon the organism in question: the person.[40] Finally in 1906, he reconciled the two outcomes of vaccination— immunity and hypersensitivity—in a new framework of altered reactivity he called allergy.[41] The modern concept of allergy grew from the study of injuries following mass administration of vaccines using the hypodermic syringe.

The prevalence of serum sickness posed a dilemma for authorities, doctors, and government. Warren Vaughan summarized this concern in his book on allergy, *Strange Malady* (1941):

> Serum disease, as this is called, is a man-made malady. If we had no curative serums and if there were no such thing as a hypodermic syringe with which to introduce the material under the skin, there would be no serum disease. Instead multitudes would still be dying from diphtheria and lockjaw and several other infections. Thus we find ourselves in somewhat of a dilemma, faced with the necessity for choosing the lesser of two potential evils.[42]

In England, there was no legal choice between the two "evils" until 1898. In the United States, mandatory vaccination laws—that included quarantine and isolation—were primarily the responsibility of state and local governments. In 1827, Boston was the first city to require smallpox vaccination for public school students. Other cities and states followed with their own mandatory vaccination laws. Legislation developed based on changes in disease and available vaccines. But the British public was uneasy about vaccination, and there were levels of noncompliance with the compulsory law—some preferred to take their chances with the disease.

Throughout much of the nineteenth century, the passive arm-to-arm technique for smallpox was used at the vaccination stations around England. Paid "vaccinators" would apply matter to multiple sites on the arms and legs of children. Since the vaccinators received a commission for every certificate of successful vaccination, they were motivated to treat as many people as possible. Aggressive vaccinators were loathed by many mothers who were fearful of the often-contaminated matter and yet were forced by law to submit their children to the treatment.[43] Mothers who refused vaccination were hunted and found. Also known as baby hunters, the government vaccinators used entrapment techniques to unearth dodgers. Parents with means, on the other hand, paid for calf lymph and the services of a doctor.[44]

As the lancet made way for the syringe, severe criticism of the perceived panacea of vaccination came from the public and some doctors in Europe and the United States. It was suggested that vaccination might actually have spread smallpox. In *Vaccine Delusion* (1898), British naturalist Alfred Wallace questioned the efficacy of vaccination. He used statistics and charts to prove that smallpox increased significantly with the administration of vaccine.

Others believed that the disease had declined as a result of improved sanitation (bedbugs were believed to carry the disease) and waste disposal protocols and natural nutrition led by health crusaders such as Sylvester Graham (1795–1851).[45] Graham was a Presbyterian minister and vegetarian who created not only a system of living but also healthful foods such as the graham cracker.

Dr. William Young in *Killed by Vaccination* (1887) objected to the "useless, cruel and inhumane law of compulsory vaccination under cover of which, as has been stated in the House of Commons, children are slaughtered by wholesale."

Socialist playwright George Bernard Shaw (1856–1950) joined the opposition to smallpox vaccination despite having nearly died from the disease in 1881.

In the 1909 preface to *The Doctor's Dilemma* (1906), he expounded on the perils of vaccination. He cited the example of Koch's 1894 tuberculin vaccine, the results of which "were not accidents, but perfectly orderly and inevitable phenomena following the injection of dangerously strong 'vaccines' at the wrong moment, and reinforcing the disease instead of stimulating the resistance to it."[46]

Shaw pointed to the process of opsonization in which an antigen is marked for destruction by a phagocyte. Antibodies, for example, will coat an antigen. The antibodies then bind to receptors on the membrane of the phagocytic cells that, in turn, ingest the antigen. This, Shaw suggested, was a concept well beyond the understanding of most doctors. Not only did doctors not understand the risks of vaccination, argued Shaw, but also they were in it for the money. Vaccines were cheap to make and lucrative in their application. And an epidemic "windfall" made the job of vaccinators and doctors even more lucrative, opined Shaw. An outbreak inspired a panic and rush for vaccination, which would then be "defended desperately were it twice as dirty, dangerous and unscientific than it is." Vaccination is not about science, but it's about economics, declared Shaw.

In 1898, the British government switched to calf lymph suspended in glycerin for a still-disconcerted public, stating that this new vaccine was purified. This improvement was perhaps a concession that paved the way for a new vaccination technique using the hypodermic syringe. The needle, however, was not much of an advance for mothers of children who began to exhibit a host of strange new reactions after injection. Serum sickness to the injected vaccine was unlike anything provoked by the vaccinator's contaminated cowpox pus. It was the first man-made allergic phenomenon created en mass in children.

DISCOVERY OF FOOD ANAPHYLAXIS

It was during his famous 1901 vaccination experiments on dogs that French immunologist Charles Richet (1850–1935) discovered what he termed *anaphylaxis*. Richet and his colleague Paul Portier were on board the yacht of oceanographer *Prince Albert I of Monaco* to explore the possibility of producing a vaccine to physalia poison, a toxin from the tentacles of the Portuguese man-of-war. The scientists began by injecting dogs with the toxin. Dogs that survived were given time to recover and then reinjected.

Richet expected that the first exposure to the poison would have created a certain amount of immunity in the dogs. Instead, the initial exposure made the dogs hypersensitive. A second much smaller dose of toxin caused a violent reaction akin to serum sickness that quickly killed the animals. In his lab, Richet soon discovered that even a small dose of proteins injected into a dog followed by another small dose several weeks later produced the same result.

This deadly reaction, Richet observed, depended not upon the dose (contrary to Von Pirquet) since even the smallest dose would trigger it, but upon the time interval between injections (similar to Von Pirquet). Further research by Nicolas Arthus in 1903 and Richard Otto in 1905 showed that without exception, all proteins considered toxic or nontoxic outside the body could produce anaphylaxis through injection—egg, milk, meat, diphtheria. And although the key again was interval, this incubation period also varied between species and between substances.

To describe this phenomenon, Richet paired two Greek words in anaphylaxis—*ana* (against) and *phylaxis* (protection)—essentially the opposite outcome they sought with vaccination.[47] In his acceptance speech for the 1913 Nobel Prize in Medicine for his work on anaphylaxis, Richet described the reaction as one of three possible outcomes of vaccination. These were the following: unchanged sensitivity or stability, diminished sensitivity or habituation, and heightened sensitivity. The first injection, instead of protecting the organism, wrote Richet, rendered it more fragile and susceptible. After an incubation period of several weeks, a second injection of the same proteins triggered anaphylaxis.[48]

Alimentary or food anaphylaxis, Richet had discovered through experiments, was the body's defensive response to proteins that had bypassed the modifying process of the digestive system and been introduced directly to the bloodstream.[49]

By injection, Richet sensitized dogs, cats, rabbits, horses, and frogs to a variety of foods, showing that the phenomenon is universal to all animals. For example, he created anaphylaxis to raw meat in dogs. Initially, he fed the animals cooked meat and measured their leucocyte or white blood cell levels that were normal. When he fed the dogs raw meat, white blood cell levels quickly increased. Richet deduced from this that "digestive juices" were required to modify the proteins of the raw meat, and if this was not accomplished, the body would mount an immune response. Subsequently, Richet injected raw meat proteins into the dogs, which provoked an anaphylactic reaction.[50] Again, in this instance, Richet created anaphylaxis in the animal through ingestion of a food combined with an injection of the same proteins. The doctor combined two functional mechanisms to achieve the condition.

Dogs, of course, eat raw meat all the time without developing anaphylaxis. At a 1913 International Medical Congress in London, Richet confirmed that it was difficult to bring about food anaphylaxis by just eating a food:

> Experimental alimentary anaphylaxis is difficult to bring about under conditions of healthy digestion, since it is a question of toxalbumins or nutritive albumins . . . because the digestive juices actively intervene in transforming these albumins and rendering them innocuous.[51]

Another aspect to anaphylaxis was the specificity in identity between the preparatory and unleashing substances. Richet identified the phenomena of cross reactivity of "allied protein groups" when he found that the injection of milk from different animals produced similar anaphylactic symptoms in a sensitized dog.

Significantly, Richet also observed that the incubation period between sensitizing and unleashing injections varied according to the substance used. A minimum period of one week between injections was indicated to create anaphylaxis to milk in a guinea pig but two weeks for mussel protein.[52]

Despite his view that anaphylaxis was universal—all animals were subject to it—Richet had little sympathy for those who acquired it through vaccination. In fact, a highly prejudicial concept of biological superiority and evolutionary socialism informed Richet's view of anaphylaxis related to vaccination. Postvaccinal anaphylaxis weeded out the weak:

> Anaphylaxis is thus necessary to the species, often to the detriment of the individual. The individual may perish, but this does not matter. The species must at all times retain its organic integrity. Anaphylaxis defends the species against the peril of adulteration.[53]

THE ORIGINS OF THE INGESTION HYPOTHESIS

Although anaphylactic reactions to sera were common among children, food anaphylaxis in a clinical setting was not. And because it was uncommon, there was a struggle to provide an in-the-field explanation for its infrequent-although-growing appearance. Literature reveals that doctors began to dismantle and boil down the landmark observations of Richet, to pick and choose bits that seemed to provide that explanation.

Doctors relied on one aspect of Richet's anaphylaxis research. Richet had stated that food sensitization occurred when proteins unmodified by the digestive system entered the blood stream. And so, ingestion of food by persons with inadequate digestion appeared to be a common sense prerequisite for food allergy. This neat explanation covered the increasing caseload of non-life-threatening food allergies, and it seemed also to fit those few cases of food anaphylaxis. At the time, anaphylactic reactions were primarily linked to egg but also to fish and dairy.[54] But Richet had combined two functional mechanisms to create food anaphylaxis—ingestion and injection. Of these two mechanisms Richet had explored in his research, injection was exorcised from the nascent ingestion hypothesis. It was assumed again that children with food anaphylaxis simply had unhealthy digestion. Nor was there much interest in other physical conditions that might contribute to individual sensitization. In fact, observed differences between animals in anaphylaxis experiments constituted "noise" rather than a signal to researchers.[55]

A problem, yet unidentified, was that the cursory and incomplete ingestion hypothesis quickly became a knee-jerk explanation even as food anaphylaxis increased through the decades. At the time, however, demand for more research on the problem was limited. Life-threatening food anaphylaxis was still relatively uncommon.

A case of "egg poisoning," in which a boy suffered from angioedema and asthma after eating the food, was reported in 1908 by English physician Alfred Schofield.[56] Another in 1912 was described as an idiosyncrasy by a New York pediatrician, Oscar Schloss. An infant at ten days of age was given raw egg white to calm diarrhea. He next ate egg at fourteen months of age at which time "he cried out, clawed at his mouth, and his tongue and mouth swelled until they were many times normal size." Schloss suggested that the boy's experience might be due to a new condition that had been receiving so much attention called allergy. To confirm his suspicions, Schloss injected the boy's blood into a guinea pig. Later he injected egg white. The animal went into anaphylactic shock.[57]

To prove anaphylaxis, doctors used injection—a dramatic and arguably unnecessary gesture. And yet, again, as a mechanism that might help explain the boy's initial sensitization, the needle was simply not considered.

Another anaphylactic food reaction was reported in "Absorption of Undigested Protein from the Alimentary Tract as Determined by the Direct Anaphylaxis Test"[58] in the *American Journal of Physiology* in 1925. The de facto conclusion in the title of the article revealed how entrenched the ingestion hypothesis had become. Injection as a mechanism of initial sensitization was not considered even as the authors of the article unleashed food anaphylaxis by injecting yet another guinea pig with blood from the egg allergic patient. An "intoxicating dose of the suspected protein (egg white) was injected intraperitoneally into the test animal, resulting in anaphylaxis." The authors did not pose the question that from the perspective of 2015 would be most salient: Why was food anaphylaxis albeit a rare condition, primarily to egg at this time? Why not to peanut, for example?

The expeditious ingestion hypothesis was handed down through twentieth-century medical literature because it explained the vast majority of food reactions. These reactions manifested not in life-threatening anaphylaxis but in a variety of uncomfortable and hard-to-diagnose symptoms such as migraines, digestive upsets, skin conditions, fatigue, anxiety, irritability, and behavioral problems.[59] As early as 1905, Dr. Francis Hare had written *The Food Factor in Disease*, a two-volume book that recommended elimination diets to help manage disease. The relationship of food sensitivity and disease appeared sporadically in medical journals such as the *Archives of Internal Medicine, Journal of the American Medical Association*, and *Annals of Clinical Medicine* in the 1920s and onward.[60] The editorial for the first 1929 issue of the US *Journal of Allergy* explained that the clinical use of the word *allergy* was to describe a broad variety of symptoms to as many substances. Anaphylaxis was reserved for those less common and violent reactions.

Vaughan's *Strange Malady* summarized the thinking about food anaphylaxis at the time. Vaughan again explained the ingestion hypothesis related to intestinal permeability that resulted in the escape of proteins into the blood stream:

> How can one become allergic to egg when nobody has ever injected egg into him? Under certain conditions egg protein taken by mouth may be absorbed undigested through the intestines and into the blood just as though it had been injected through the skin. A period of indigestion, some vitamin deficiency favoring abnormal absorption, overeating, temporary disturbance in the activity of the digestive juices, or some other factor might promote absorption of undigested protein.[61]

Vaughan assumed that egg proteins had never been injected—and he may have been correct, but it seems not to have been investigated as even a possible mechanism of sensitization. In one sentence, the doctor removed injection from the discussion of anaphylaxis altogether. And yet, emulsified egg lecithin had been used extensively in vaccines prior to the publication of Vaughan's book. In 1931, vaccine manufacturers had introduced fertile hen's egg as a medium for growing viruses. This was seen as an advance because vaccines grown on mouse brain had produced allergic brain encephalitis in some children.[62] Vaughan, however, stated that adverse vaccine reactions, including serum sickness, had all but vanished in 1941 due to the improvements in "purifying serums."[63]

Vaughan was satisfied to focus on consumption as the sole cause of sensitization even in babies in utero. He pointed to mothers whose "abnormal food cravings" during pregnancy might cause sensitization. The doctor did not see the problem in his logic when he stated that food anaphylaxis is an "abnormal" reaction *primarily* to egg. If anaphylaxis was almost always to egg, how could it be abnormal?

Something linked the egg-allergic patients. Again, why egg and not beef or pork or any of the thousands of common proteins children and mothers ate at this time—including peanuts, an inexpensive staple in US households? Peanut allergy appears not to have been a concern at this time. Vaughan mentions peanuts once in his book but as a crushed topping and nothing more. Among the foods to which people had developed allergies and anaphylaxis, peanut was not one of them. How and why was egg an anaphylactic concern for children and peanut was not? Injection as a mechanism for sensitization or even as a contributing factor still did not feature in the medical literature even as doctors explored "antianaphylaxis" injection treatments.

Like trying to put the genie back in the bottle, early allergists used repeated "subanaphylactic" doses of substances to desensitize allergy sufferers. Jay Schamberg had observed in 1919 that tolerance to poison ivy in Native American populations was achieved through the preventive practice of chewing poison ivy shoots. Richard Otto contended that the anaphylactic antibody might become exhausted or neutralized by injections of the substances to which one was allergic. However, these injections proved to be a temporary reprieve for most and tended to provoke anaphylactic reactions.[64]

And so, the incomplete ingestion hypothesis persisted as a blanket explanation for food anaphylaxis. And it remained so even during the first outbreak of food anaphylaxis that occurred to one food starting in the late 1930s. Literature revealed a sudden surge in anaphylaxis to cottonseed oil in the United States that peaked in the 1940s and dissipated through the '50s.

THE FIRST OUTBREAK OF FOOD ANAPHYLAXIS

Research in clinical allergy grew slowly and not at all in anaphylaxis. Infectious disease continued to dominate the attention of doctors and pharmaceutical companies. Great strides were made during World War II in the development of injected antibiotics. This "wonder drug" developed in 1928 by Scottish-born biologist Alexander Fleming (1881–1955) promised cures for all manner of infections from gonorrhea to tonsillitis. But it was during World War II for treatment of wounded soldiers that solutions were found to mass production of the drug. In 1942, the Pfizer Company in Brooklyn, New York, emerged as the leader in the mass production of penicillin because of its historical expertise in fermentation. By 1944, this and other companies had met the demand for the injected drug that included a homegrown oil excipient, refined cottonseed oil.[65] Cottonseed oil was used in the delivery of both injected and oral penicillin. A novel solution to the rapid excretion of injected penicillin by the kidneys—one dose would last only a few hours—was created in 1945 by Dr. Raymond Libby of the American Cyanamide Company. The doctor suspended the drug in cotton-seed oil and sealed them in a gelatin capsule.[66] The cottonseed oil and drug were not released until the capsule—bypassing the modifying effects of many digestive enzymes, including stomach acids—finally reached the small intestines.

Before World War II, experiments with food oil excipients in vaccines included oil from castor bean, cottonseed, corn, olives, and more. Starting as early as 1913, these oils were often emulsified with hydrolyzed casein (dairy protein) or egg lecithin.[67] An emulsion is a mixture of two or more immiscible liquids. One liquid is dispersed in another; the most common being oil and water into which a surface active substance can increase the stability of the mixture so that it can be stored for lengthy periods.

Yanol produced in Japan, for example, was an emulsion made from 3% castoreum (oil secreted by beavers) and stabilized by egg lecithin. Tested in the United States in the 1930s, this product had to be withdrawn due to side effects such as shaking fits, fever, and anaphylaxis. In the 1940s, a second generation of fat emulsions emerged. One of the best known on the market under the name

Lipomul introduced in 1935 and marketed in the '40s was made with refined cottonseed oil.

The process of refining the oil for use in these excipients was crucial. This process removed proteins from the oil, well known by this time to cause allergic sensitization if injected. As it was, many side effects occurred with cottonseed oil such as vomiting, shaking fits, tachycardia, drop in blood pressure, difficulties breathing, and shock.[68] Cottonseed oil contains the toxic steroid gossypol, which later became a common agricultural pesticide.

Concerns regarding the "anaphylactogenic potency" of cottonseed oil emerged before 1943.[69] Warren Vaughan warned cottonseed-allergic readers to be aware of this hidden ingredient in many processed foods, including mayonnaise, vegetable shortening, and canned tuna.[70] Sensitivity to cottonseed oil grew through the 1930s and was still a significant concern in 1950.[71]

In 1947, worries over the spread of cottonseed allergy evident through increasing allergic reactions to it in processed foods were taken to a committee at the US Federal Security Agency. Testimony given before the agency was published in a 1949 report. At the inquiry, two out of six doctors challenged the assertion that refined cottonseed oil was actually free from allergenic proteins.[72] Testimony from oil-processing technicians revealed that the machinery used for the commercial refining of cottonseed oil was not thoroughly cleaned before it was used for the refining of another oil. These sloppy procedures, it was suggested, had led to the contamination of various oils with cottonseed oil.[73] It was suggested that this hidden contaminant had resulted in an outbreak of anaphylactic reactions. None, though, ventured to inquire into the causes of initial sensitization. How were these people made allergic to cottonseed oil in the first place?

While the Association of Cottonseed Products argued that food labels did not need to list the refined oil because it was free of allergens, suspicion remained regarding the quality of cottonseed oil. An explanation for the inconsistency in the quality of the oil and the resulting cross-contamination may have begun with a challenged cottonseed industry weakened by bad deals, bad luck, and the Depression. Between 1909 and 1920, a boll weevil blight saw the price of cotton tumble from ¢34.98 per pound in 1919 to ¢9.4 per pound, causing the agricultural crisis of 1920–21. The Crash of 1929 and drought from 1929–39 forced many cotton farmers from the land. The number of cotton farms fell from 123,477 to 86,889 in Oklahoma alone and harvested acreage decreased dramatically from over 4 million to 1.6 million. Declining production marked the industry for the remainder of the twentieth century.[74]

Adding to this misery was a conflict over seed grading between the Cottonseed Crushers' Association and the federal government, the United States Department of Agriculture (USDA). In 1930–31, attempts to come to an agreement were stalled when a Federal Trade Commission found rule violations. In addition, 1930s New Deal acreage allotments reduced cottonseed yields. As a result of these challenges, the availability of cottonseed oil began to diminish.

By the late '40s, cottonseed oil was demoted to minor product in the competitive food oils industry,[75] and it was largely but not entirely replaced in the delivery of vaccines and drugs. At the same time, the prevalence of cottonseed anaphylaxis fell. Intense interest in this allergy in the 1940s dropped sharply through the 1950s. Infrequent titles appear subsequently in the medical literature with an unusual report of "new concerns over an old problem" with the brief reemergence of several cases of cottonseed allergy in the late 1980s.[76] Cottonseed oil proteins are considered potent allergens. In refining processes in the 2000s, the presence of any cottonseed oil proteins in other refined oils violated the specifications of the US Pharmacopoeia (USP).[77]

In choosing a vegetable oil replacement for the unreliable cottonseed oil at the close of World War II, US vaccine makers chose one that was tariff protected, cheap, abundant, and homegrown—its wide availability had made it an important source of glycerin in the manufacture of explosives during the two world wars.

After World War II, the all-American peanut replaced cottonseed as the oil ingredient of choice in the manufacture of penicillin and later in vaccines.[78]

Chapter 5

THE HISTORY OF PEANUT ALLERGY

PEANUT OIL IN PENICILLIN: NOT THE 'SMOKING GUN'

In Queens, New York, during the summer of 1943, two-year-old Patricia Malone was dying. She had been diagnosed with acute staphylococcic septicemia, a bacteria that had left her delirious and barely breathing. On August 15 at 3:40 p.m., the city editor of the *New York Journal–American* received a call from the child's father. She had only seven hours to live unless she received the new drug called penicillin.

Penicillin was difficult to obtain and make in large quantities. It took a chemist a whole day to produce just one small flask of it. And even then, one dose of the wonder drug would last for just three hours before being excreted by the kidneys. Worse yet, penicillin was under severe restrictions during the war. The only man authorized to release the antibiotic to civilians was Dr. Chester Keffer in Boston. Through a series of frantic calls and telegrams, Keffer was persuaded to authorize the release of a quantity of the drug from Squibb Labs in New Brunswick, New Jersey. A police escort raced with the dying child's doctor to the lab where they obtained the drug and rushed back to the city. After two days on an intravenous penicillin drip, the child was dramatically improved. In six weeks she was back home.[1]

Mass production was one of the main obstacles to the widespread use of penicillin. This problem was solved in time for the D-day invasion thanks to a process of deep-tank fermentation devised by a small Brooklyn, New York, company, Charles Pfizer & Company, and a chemical engineer named Jasper Kane. In March 1943, Kane began experimenting with 147,500-gallon tanks, and by the end of the year the company had mass produced over forty-five million units of penicillin. On June 6, 1944, 90% of allied soldiers were carrying a dose of the antibiotic produced in Brooklyn.[2]

The second significant obstacle to the mass application of penicillin was the short-term effect of a single dose. In 1945, penicillin pioneer Alexander Fleming (1881–1955) was touring the US Walter Reed Army Medical Center where virtually every soldier had been injected with penicillin. While there, Fleming learned of two army doctors who had solved the dose duration problem by administering injected penicillin in a mixture of peanut oil and beeswax.

US Army Medical Corps Captain Monroe J. Romansky (1911–2006) had discovered a method of prolonging the action of penicillin by mixing it with 4% to 4.8% beeswax and peanut oil to create POB (penicillin in oil beeswax) also known as the Romansky formula.[3] The mix was a viscous, butterlike substance that was difficult to draw up into the syringe.[4]

It was a simple solution to the problem. The peanut oil in the POB coated the penicillin particles. As the body metabolized the wax and oil, the drug was released slowly into the system. The formula extended the dose from three hours to single daily injections. This sustained release with peanut oil, however, was not new. Since at least 1940, allergists had started using a commercial brand of epinephrine in peanut oil to control "intractable asthma."[5] Although there were "records of unusual reactions to this preparation," including urticaria (hives), Romansky's use of peanut oil became a standard in the manufacture of penicillin from that desperate wartime moment on. For his innovation, President Truman awarded the doctor the Legion of Merit.

Penicillin POB actually doubled penicillin blood levels according to research at the Montreal General Hospital in 1947. But this success was not without side effects. The amount of beeswax and oil used was reduced "in an attempt to eliminate undesirable reactions."[6] And in 1950, a study of penicillin treatments in over one hundred children at the Philadelphia Children's Hospital reported additional obstacles to the formula. The Romansky formula had created peanut allergy in an undisclosed number of children:

Although good clinical results were reported, certain disadvantages were encountered, namely, difficulty in administration, variability of absorption, local pain at the site of injection, sensitivity to peanut oil or beeswax, and sterile abscess formation.[7]

Iatrogenic side effects, including allergy from penicillin injections, were "distinct hazards."[8] And urticaria was a significant side effect of POB. Because of this, doctors at the World Health Organization were alarmed at the overuse and misuse of the drug. In 1953, six hundred tons of penicillin, streptomycin, and broad-spectrum antibiotics were produced.[9] Their widespread application had resulted in fatal anaphylaxis, antibiotic-resistant bacterial strains, fungal overgrowth, and gastrointestinal dysbiosis.[10]

An estimated 2.5% of all children injected with penicillin developed an allergy to it.

In 1948, doctors F. H. Buckwalter and H. L. Dickison also began to use penicillin with aluminum monostearate (PAM), an aqueous solution again suspended in peanut oil with aluminum monostearate. PAM was much easier to administer than POB, and it produced desirable penicillin blood levels for twenty-four to twenty-six hours. PAM was recommended by the WHO for control of syphilis, yaws (a tropical infection of bones and joints caused by spirochete bacterium), and other infections. By the end of 1957, approximately thirty-five million people had been injected with the peanut oil based PAM.[11] PAM continued to be commonly used through the 1960s, 1970s, and 1980s.[12]

Allergic reactivity, including anaphylaxis, emerged during what was called the PAM era. The incidence and severity of reactions to PAM increased significantly over those experienced with POB. For at least one doctor, the mass allergic reactions to penicillin reminded him of "serum sickness of former days."[13] In 1953, the media warned of increased "peril" from penicillin. Severe and fatal anaphylactoid reactions were being reported with increasing frequency.[14] In a study of 1,200 syphilitic patients at the Royal Victoria Hospital in Montreal, 12% of patients reacted with allergic symptoms to penicillin.

In essence, the use of penicillin had created a mass allergic phenomenon with anaphylactic fatalities.[15] And since the United States had the highest rate of consumption of penicillin in the world at this time, the majority of fatalities to the drug were reported there. Between 1% and 10% of the US population was allergic to penicillin in 2009—the wide range attributed to insufficient formal study yielding to anecdotal reports.

It was important that the peanut oil used in penicillin was refined to remove as much of the sensitizing peanut proteins as possible. However, not only was it impossible to remove all the proteins,[16] but also the quality of refinement varied between makers.[17] On this basis in 2000, an expert committee on labeling at the WHO resisted giving a full endorsement to the oil.[18] Investigations had shown that refined peanut oil in foods had both sensitized and caused allergic reactions in children.[19] Refined peanut oil can create allergy whether consumed or injected.

It is reasonable to expect that a number of people injected with POB or PAM became peanut allergic. While statistics do not exist for peanut allergy from this time, a study published in 2010 asked people born during this period whether they had peanut or nut allergies. And while it is not known when those polled acquired their allergies, 0.3% of people born between 1944–47, 0.4% born between 1948–57, and 0.6% born between 1959–67 reported having a peanut allergy.[20] When asked in 2008, over 1% of people born during this period, 1944–67, reported an allergy to any nut, including peanut. It is important to emphasize that in 1941, allergist Warren Vaughan saw a variety of food allergies, many to egg and dairy, but none to peanut in either child or adult. By the later '40s and '50s, it would be expected that peanut allergy would have cut across all demographics. Penicillin was administered to adults and children alike. The medical literature indicates that peanut allergy drew increasing interest from doctors through the 1960s. The first formal US study of peanut allergy in children was finally launched in 1973. Peanut allergy emerged for the first time as a growing if minor concern for children.

During the late '40s and '50s, peanut oil in penicillin appeared to be relatively safe, and so it acquired a history of acceptable use. It became a reasonable choice for inclusion in many other injectable drugs.[21] It continued to be used as a base for injected epinephrine for children with asthma,[22] in anesthetics, and as an adjuvant in vaccines for tetanus at this time.[23] It was used in oral drugs.[24] Unknown to the consumer, refined peanut oil became a popular ingredient in injected and oral medications, vitamins, skin creams, infant formula, and more.[25]

WHY PEANUT?

Peanut oil was a natural choice for Romansky during World War II. Peanuts were homegrown, tariff protected, relatively inexpensive, plentiful, remained stable in heat for long periods without going rancid,[26] and above all, they were not rationed during the war. During war and in times of scarcity—the Civil War, both world wars, and the Great Depression—Americans had turned to peanut and peanut oil as substitutes for food, medicine, and fuel. And it should be noted that during none of these difficult times with heavy peanut consumption did there appear to be any issues with peanut and allergy. It just didn't seem to exist.

Romansky had few oils from which to choose in creating his penicillin formulation. All imports of oil (especially coconut oil, which was most stable in heat) from the Philippines and British colonies in Asia were cut off after the bombing of Pearl Harbor. And cottonseed oil, the only other contender for homegrown excipient that had been a favorite before the war, was unreliable. There was suspicion that refined cottonseed oil being produced at the time was not free of sensitizing proteins and that it was toxic.

The cottonseed industry had been weakened by bad deals and bad luck. As previously discussed, the 1909–1920 boll weevil blight that precipitated an agricultural crisis in 1919 was only the beginning of the misfortune for cottonseed. The Crash of 1929 was followed by a drought from 1929–39 that forced cotton farmers from the land. When they did return, it was to grow peanuts. Peanuts were suited to the same soil as cotton and appeared more resistant to insects.

During the US Civil War when the northern blockade prevented the import of goods by the South, peanut and peanut oil were used as substitutes for innumerable essentials. Peanut oil was a superior replacement for whale oil to lubricate machinery because it didn't smoke.[27] It was used extensively as a lubricant for railroad locomotives, wood, and cotton spindles. Cooks substituted peanut oil for lard—lard, especially from pork, was the preferred frying medium in the United States. In fact, pigs were fed peanut and allowed to run in the fields to route them up.[28] Confederacy Army cooks used peanuts extensively in cooking as malnutrition and hunger persisted through the war. Peanuts were substituted for coffee and were used as recipe fillers. Recipes were created for peanut drinks, peanut pie, peanut sausage, and peanut mayonnaise.

But as the Civil War ended, so too did the large-scale emergency manufacture of peanut oil. Attempts to reignite the peanut industry postwar were not wholly successful, and the limited demand for the oil was satisfied by German imports made from peanuts grown in their African colonies. With the outbreak of another war, World War I, this import from Germany ceased.

At the same time, however, the demand for peanut oil skyrocketed. Peanut, the wartime substitute, was needed even more desperately in the form of glycerin when the United States entered World War I in 1917. Glycerin was used to make explosives. To meet the sudden demand, peanut oil mills sprang up throughout the South, and cultivation of the legume increased to four million acres, on land formerly used for cotton.

In the United States, peanuts became closely aligned with war. They were so much a part of wartime that eating and growing them became patriotic acts. "Peanuts and Patriotism," a 1917 article in *The Forum,* exclaimed that peanuts served valiantly in the war effort by conserving dairy products, substituting for meat and feeding livestock.[29] And the National Emergency Food Garden Commission encouraged even small gardeners to grow them.

During the Great War, peanuts became one of the most important commercial crops in the United States. But with the close of the war, cheap peanut imports flooded the United States and domestic prices plummeted. Needing government intervention to regain control of the market, a suffering peanut industry turned to the influential agricultural chemist George Washington Carver (1864–1943).

Carver knew of 30,117 uses for peanut.[30] He had developed a host of products with peanut—including axle grease, adhesives, cosmetics, linoleum, metal polish, shaving cream, wood stain, and a vitalizing skin rub for polio victims.[31] Carver patented several of his peanut discoveries, including a formula for Penol. Penol was cough syrup made from an emulsion of peanut juices and creosote.

In 1921, Carver was asked to speak as an expert witness before the House Ways and Means Committee on behalf of the United Peanut Growers' Association. The group was seeking tariff protection from the flood of peanuts and peanut oil coming from China and Japan. At the hearing, Carver began by presenting his Pandora's box filled with 101 peanut products.[32] Initially allotted only ten minutes, Carver spoke for an hour and forty minutes as he presented peanut candies, cakes, peanut "milk," mock meats, breakfast foods, shoe polish, and wood stains. The committee applauded his valuable contributions to science. At his second presentation to the Finance Committee, Carver's plea on behalf of the peanut industry was successful. With a tariff in place, peanut imports began to decline.

This tariff protection set the peanut industry up for a boom, and World War II created the opportunity for it to happen. During this war, the per capita consumption of peanuts and peanut products almost doubled due to shortages of other foods, the nonrationing of peanuts, and lack of competition from imported and domestic nuts and oils. In 1942, *Fortune Magazine* claimed that six hundred million pounds of peanut oil would need to be produced for food and, again in wartime, for glycerin in the manufacture of explosives.[33] The secretary of agriculture launched the Food for Freedom program in 1943, telling farmers they needed to plant 5.5 million acres of peanuts. The peanut could win the war and sustain them in peacetime.[34]

Through World War II, the peanut industry doubled in size, and prices were two to three times higher than before the war. By 1944, twice as much land was utilized than before the war to produce 2.5 billion pounds of peanuts worth $200,000,000.[35] The equivalent in 2009 would be about $24.5 billion.

Determined that this boom in peanut sales would not end, the US National Peanut Council threw money at increasing public consumption of the legume. The council proposed to spend $1,000,000 over three years to find new uses for the peanut, to study insect infestation control, and to promote the peanut's role in American life. Industry leaders were also concerned that the government market protections might be eliminated. Although the industry had never been stronger and it was reported that Americans ate more peanuts than any other people, the council president Walter Richards stated, "Our present situation is dangerous and may lead to a serious crisis."[36]

By January 1945, a reporter from *The New York Times* wrote that a shortage of peanuts loomed. And in October 1945, the retail prices of peanut butter increased by ¢6 per pound. The Peanut and Nut Salters Association warned of a shortage of civilian supplies of peanut predicting a 50% cut.[37] But the fears were unfounded. By 1947, there was a "whopper" crop, and exports had climbed to 45% of the total peanut market.[38] Government-subsidized grants and loans had helped cushion the transition from wartime to peacetime.[39] In 1950, 2,200,000 acres were allotted to this crop producing two billion pounds of peanuts.[40]

Peanut oil in the manufacture of penicillin POB was an easy choice for Romansky during World War II. It was available during wartime, stable in heat, relatively inexpensive, and patriotic. And again, while the exact number of people made peanut allergic are unknown for the postwar years, this minor allergy would have cut across all demographics. Injected penicillin was administered to adults and children alike.

Articles published in 1956, 1961, and 1963[41] reflected a growing awareness of the allergy in medical circles, but there was no impact from this on public consumption or on peanut industry revenues. In fact, the peanut industry continued to experience growth. In the 1970s, the unprecedented demand following the election of peanut farmer President Jimmy Carter (1977–81) was like winning the lottery. The themed presidency of "Peanut One" spurred soaring consumption of peanuts and peanut butter in schools and a bonanza for growers.[42] Testament to power of the peanut industry was the continued support of government when the 1995 Farm Bill challenged farmer subsidies. Peanut-friendly government representatives ensured that supply management was again secured in law for the all-American crop.[43]

The peanut industry remained strong until a marked decline in the 1990s when the peanut-allergy epidemic took a bite out of its bottom line. Between 1993 and 1999, the peanut's share of the snack foods market fell from 14.4% to 12.4%.[44] Of a $21.6 billion industry in 2006, this drop represented a significant loss[45] of about $432 million in annual gross revenues. The important consumer category of children under fourteen was in decline.

VACCINE ADJUVANTS & ALLERGY: THE IMMUNOLOGIST'S DIRTY SECRET

In 1964, *The New York Times*[46] announced that pharmaceutical giant Merck had begun to use a new vaccine ingredient that promised to extend immunity against influenza, polio, and other illnesses.[47] This new ingredient patented just four days earlier was called Adjuvant 65-4.[48] It contained up to 65% peanut oil as well as Arlacel A, aluminum stearate, and other ingredients. The *Times* article explained the impressive value of the peanut oil in the adjuvant that was similar to its action in penicillin. The oil surrounds the vaccine antigens. When the vaccine is injected into the muscle, the oil is gradually metabolized by the body providing a sustained release of the other ingredients.[49]

Adjuvant 65 had been a six-year research effort between Merck and the Children's Hospital of Philadelphia, the same hospital in which experiments using the Romansky formula on children had resulted in peanut allergies. In 1966, Merck introduced this novel peanut oil additive to the public in a flu vaccine.[50]

An adjuvant (from the Latin *adjuvare* [to enhance]) is a vaccine additive that stimulates the body's production of antibodies to a viral or bacterial antigen. In the 1930s, American immunologist Jules Freund (1890–1960) created an adjuvant by mixing aluminum mineral salts with mycobacteria in emulsified mineral oil.[51] Freund's complete adjuvant (FCA) was quickly withdrawn, however, and banned from use in humans because of its toxic side effects. FCA produced granulomas, abscesses, and autoimmune diseases. According to writer Gary Matsumoto, Freund himself had warned that animals injected with his adjuvant developed severe allergic conditions such as allergic aspermatogenesis (loss of sperm production), experimental allergic encephalomyelitis (MS), and allergic neuritis (leading to paralysis). The oil-in-water emulsion without added mycobacteria is known as Freund's incomplete adjuvant (FIA) and, being less toxic, was used in human vaccines. Mineral oil adjuvants are no longer used in humans in the United States and many other countries.

Thus the arrival of Adjuvant 65 meant hope for the creation of safer and more widely distributed vaccines. Previous experiments with other adjuvants in flu vaccines had had limited success. In a 1964, British study of over nine hundred subjects (allergic subjects were excluded) shot with a flu vaccine, one subject was incapacitated, and several others actually developed the flu, resulting in consumer resistance to the products.[52] These vaccine designs did not, as was hoped, incite a "desire for revaccination."

Next to such failures, the introduction of Adjuvant 65-4 in a flu vaccine in the late 1960s was seen as an improvement.[53] Several medical journal articles published in the early 1970s extolled the effectiveness of this peanut oil adjuvant that produced extremely high antibody levels. The adjuvant showed a level of antibodies that was thirteenfold higher than that produced by an aqueous medium.[54]

Adjuvant 65 had the potential to become an important addition to any vaccine. One of its inventors who had patented Adjuvant 65 with Merck, Maurice Hilleman (1919–2005),[55] helped write a report as a member of the WHO Scientific Group on Immunological Adjuvants. The report published in 1973 explained that this peanut oil with aluminum adjuvant had resulted in elevated antibody titres, elevated titers for sustained periods, a broad antigenic response, and reduced cost of production because adjuvants were antigen sparing. With an adjuvant, vaccines needed less of the expensive antigen to achieve a superior stimulation of the immune system. In addition, vegetable oil was easier to metabolize than mineral oil.[56] The mineral oil adjuvant "potentiates allergic responses."[57]

But so too could Adjuvant 65.

Hilleman and the expert group knew of the danger of injected proteins. The group conceded that any breakage of the peanut emulsions in the body, "especially when allergens are employed," was dangerous. As well it was important with oil adjuvants that the injection be administered deep into the muscle "since there is a far greater chance of adverse effects when they are deposited subcutaneously." Doctors and nurses must be carefully trained, they warned, in the art of deep muscular injection and that "they should appreciate the need for it in this context."[58]

Injection into the bloodstream would virtually guarantee allergic sensitization to peanut or any other extant vaccine proteins.

Noting that Adjuvant 65 was prepared using "highly refined arachis oil" and that within two months it was almost completely metabolized, the chance of any harmful effects was reduced. The report confirmed that "no sensitization to the components of the adjuvant, including peanut oil, occurred."

Hilleman and his colleagues knew that allergic sensitization to the peanut oil in this adjuvant was a distinct possibility. Again, it was impossible to remove all protein from peanut oil. According to the FDA, the amount of peanut protein in the refined oil varied by manufacturer, processes used, and by tests used to detect it. Trace levels of intact proteins would always remain.[59]

The Romansky formula POB and PAM had created peanut allergy. And as it turned out, oil-in-water adjuvants like Adjuvant 65, too, could create allergy to extant "contaminant proteins" in flu vaccines.

In 1973, an article on the role of a peanut oil adjuvant in flu vaccines was specifically observed to create "untoward" hypersensitivity to the proteins in the vaccine.[60] Adjuvants were hard to control in the body and caused delayed hyper-sensitivity reactions. "Trouble" lay with the oils and emulsifiers being "insufficiently characterized," stated one researcher:

> An adjuvant will indiscriminately augment immune reactions, particularly delayed hypersensitivity reactions, against all the contaminant proteins and lipo-proteins as well as against the virus antigens.[61]

Tension existed between reports prepared by Hilleman at the WHO and those in the medical literature regarding the relative safety of adjuvants. Mounting concerns in the medical literature regarding allergy echoed those expressed in the media following one of the first profiled peanut allergy deaths in the United States. In 1972, a child in Boston died after eating peanut butter ice cream.

Doctors acknowledged the rising prevalence of peanut allergy. In 1973, S. A. Bock began the first US study of 114 peanut-allergic children. By 1974, the peanut-oil-based Adjuvant 65 was licensed for general use in the United Kingdom[62] but had failed to obtain approval in the United States. And so Hilleman helped develop several other patented formulations of the same basic adjuvant attempting to satisfy government requirements.[63] It appeared that what made it effective, certain "undefined impurities," was blocking its approval. In the United States, the only stand-alone adjuvant approved by the FDA was aluminum salt (alum). The policy of the FDA was to approve adjuvants as they appeared within a complete vaccine formula. Vaccine formulae could be approved and patented with peanut-oil adjuvants but not with Adjuvant 65 as a stand-alone product.

Ultimately, the company decided not to pursue Adjuvant 65 any further in the United States.[64] According to one author, a subsequent review of the safety of Adjuvant 65 over ten years published in 1973 showed that Arlacel A in the emulsified peanut-oil adjuvant appeared to induce tumors in mice. Some believed that it was this adverse effect that had kept the formula from receiving license.[65]

Extreme caution followed the introduction of the water-in-oil aluminum adjuvants. The mechanism for alum's tendency to stimulate eosinophilia and enhance IgE production was unknown, but its consequence was an undeniable increase in allergenicity and neurotoxicity.[66] A seminal review of adjuvanted vaccines in 1980 warned that these and future vaccine additives should not risk induction of allergy or other iatrogenic illnesses.[67]

The challenge in vaccine adjuvant design was to gain potency while minimizing toxicity.[68] But many doctors saw toxicity and allergenicity as inevitable and therefore acceptable compromises in vaccination goals. In a student textbook published in 2000, one author was critical of a colleague who believed that "any toxicity that we accept is a compromise." This compromise, stated the author, "must become an accepted principle in the search for adjuvants suitable for use in human vaccines because one of their functions is to stimulate antigen presenting cells."[69]

In the late 1970s and 1980s, Adjuvant 65 was not eligible for use in US vaccines. However, it did become a model for other adjuvants. Based on Hilleman's precedent setting formula, one researcher published on a novel lipid emulsion adjuvant using peanut oil for use in humans.[70] As well, Adjuvant 65 was a precedent cited in many vaccine patents using emulsified peanut-oil adjuvants. The inclusion of peanut oil in vaccine adjuvant patents became common practice.[71] However, with the sharp rise in lawsuits against vaccine makers starting in the mid-1970s, public knowledge of exact ingredients in vaccines or other pediatric injections became circumscribed. Vaccine makers no longer excitedly announced new ingredients as Merck did in 1964 with the peanut-oil-based Adjuvant 65-4. The public had no way of knowing fully what was being injected into their children.

Adjuvants, revealed immunologist Charles Janeway (1943–2003), a Howard Hughes Medical Institute investigator and Yale University School of Medicine professor in 1989, were the "immunologists' dirty little secret." The secret was really a poorly understood puzzle regarding the body's response to them.[72] Janeway suggested that there were cross-reactive combinations of which researchers were unaware but which the body recognized.[73]

The difficult balance between potency and safety had long been recognized in vaccine design. In fact, a competitive edge between vaccine makers had been found on either side of the issues of efficacy and side effects.

CEO of BioVant Stephen Simes was quoted in a 2006 business article. In the article, the CEO was quoted as distinguishing his company's products from those of its competitors in the vaccine market based on their lower rate of allergy-inducing side effects. He was quoted to have said that the problem with most adjuvants was that they could cause allergies, and those of BioVant brand, while not as potent as others, were safer.[74] It was an unusual disclosure but one intended to boost his company's sales.

Vaccination is designed to provoke the immune system which invariably leads to the creation of IgE antibodies and the risk of permanent allergy or anaphylaxis. And peanut, as discussed in chapter 3, is more allergenic than other substances. It has been suggested that the peanut has adjuvant properties of its own that make it "a perfect allergen."[75] The "hydrophobic" residues of the amino acids in Ara h 1 peanut epitope are protected within the structure of the protein from degradation by digestion.[76] Indeed, an "allergenic" feature of proteins is their stability when heated or processed.

But the question regarding the specific sensitizing or cross-sensitizing ingredients in pediatric injections was difficult to answer after the mid-1970s. Did peanut continue to be an ingredient in these injections? Patents for a variety of pediatric vaccines include peanut oil as a possible ingredient but a patent does not mean the vaccine was produced. Or was there a homologous sensitizing protein such as castor bean oil, soybean lecithin, or even chiten in the latex rubber stopper of the syringe that cross-reacted to peanut when the food was consumed? Vaccines by design are intended to provoke the immune system—

the evolved defenses of immunity and allergy. Their twin relationship has been well described for over 100 years.

All that was clear was that peanut allergy first emerged during the later 1940s with the introduction of Romansky's peanut oil and beeswax formula in penicillin followed by PAM, penicillin in peanut oil in aluminum monostearate starting in the 1950s through the 1980s. A small but growing prevalence of the allergy came with the use of peanut oil in a range of pharmaceuticals both oral and injected, including the Adjuvant 65-4 and the use of aluminum in vaccines designed to provoke a strong immune response not only to the vaccine ingredients but also to what was in the body or environment at the time of vaccination. Peanut-allergy studies were launched in the 1970s followed by sporadic deaths from peanut allergy and increasing media attention.

And so doctors watched the slowly rising prevalence of peanut allergy, none publicly posing the obvious questions—like the cottonseed oil mystery of the 1930s and '40s, how were people being sensitized to this food in the first place? And certainly, none asked whether there had been a precedent for mass allergy in children. There was an amnesiac gap in medical memory less than 60 years old reaching back to Richet's Nobel Prize win of 1913 and his understanding of the role of vaccination in the creation of food anaphylaxis. This history would have been an important clue to causation given that peanut allergy had a significant and specific impact on children starting around 1990.

LAUNCHING THE PEANUT ALLERGY EPIDEMIC (1988-1994)

In the early 1990s, a sudden surge of peanut-allergic four- and five-year-old children filled school systems across Canada, the United Kingdom, and the United States and Australia. It caught many educators off guard.[77] Eyewitness accounts of this phenomenon confirmed by ER admission records, and two UK studies of preschoolers point to this moment—prevalence of peanut allergy in children suddenly accelerated between 1988 and 1994.

Functionally, there are a limited number of ways in which a person can become anaphylactic to any substance—through ingestion, inhalation, through broken skin, and injection. And historically, the only mechanism implicated in sudden mass allergy—from serum sickness to penicillin—was injection. Further, this period of allergy acceleration in children correlated to an unprecedented series of political, social, legal, and economic reforms directed at vaccinations.

Swift, identical alterations to the pediatric vaccination schedules of Canada, the United Kingdom, the United States, Australia, a few other Western countries occurred simultaneously between the late 1980s and early 1990s.

The peanut-allergy epidemic in children was precipitated by childhood injections. Events leading up to it unfolded in plain sight.

US Vaccine Injury Act creates liability free environment for vaccine makers

In the spring of 1985, 231 lawsuits were pending in the United States against four vaccine manufacturers.[78] Vaccine makers were paying out millions of dollars in settlements, their legal defense costs soared, and insurance was becoming prohibitive. Previously, courts had declared that vaccine makers could not be held strictly liable for selling products "with a known but apparently reasonable risk."[79] The doctors and parents were deemed largely responsible for the risk and any ensuing damage. But as injuries mounted, suits against manufacturers were allowed based on a "failure to warn." During the flu nonepidemic of 1976, emergency vaccines administered to about forty-five million people over three months were linked to a significant rise in Guillain-Barré syndrome.[80] These and other side effects resulted in more than four thousand complaints settled by the US government for $72 million.[81]

This event opened the door to a flood of vaccine-related lawsuits—cases involving the DPT vaccine escalated from one suit in 1979 to 255 in 1986. Vaccine maker Lederle estimated that total sales of its 1983 polio vaccine were only one-twelfth the value of claims filed against it.[82]

In this litigious environment many pharmaceutical companies simply abandoned the vaccine market, leaving the US supply in the hands of a few makers. Even the pharmaceutical giant Merck was challenged in 1979 by an internal report questioning their continued presence in vaccine research and development.[83] By 1985, the United States was facing a vaccine shortage that threatened public health, declared a report published by the US Institute of Medicine (IOM).[84]

To reduce the uncertainty faced by manufacturers, the IOM called for the federal government to provide "equitable, rapid compensation in a consistent fashion." In 1986, President Reagan signed the National Childhood Vaccine Injury Act from which emerged the Vaccine Injury Compensation Program (VICP) in 1988. VICP was a "no-fault" alternative to the tort system in which eligible claims would be determined by a federal court and paid by the federal government.[85] Until parents had first exhausted this approach, their tort claims could not proceed. In this new legal environment, the pressures on vaccine makers eased.[86] The number of pending lawsuits quickly dropped to just a handful.

Sudden increase in vaccination coverage rates

But US public health was perceived to be in danger from yet another source: parents who were slow to vaccinate their children before the start of school. The vaccination rate for preschool children under four years of age in 1985 was between 55% and 65%.[87] Obstacles to vaccination were cost for many but inconvenience for more: there were seven vaccines in 1985. The schedule included two combination vaccines, measles-mumps-rubella (MMR), and diphtheria-pertussis-tetanus (DPT) plus a multistrain oral polio vaccine (OPV). Parents typically put off vaccination until their children reached school-age, by which time and with school requirements, 90% of all children were fully vaccinated.

Therefore in 1991, the Bush government took action on a goal of raising national vaccination levels among preschool children to 90% by the year 2000. Vaccination action plans were formulated by all states and twenty-eight metropolitan areas. Federal grant funds were authorized for direct delivery of vaccination services as well as vaccine purchase. New awards for state grants tripled from $37 million in 1991 to $98.2 million in 1993.

The US strategy focused on preschool children was on course with the World Health Organization's 1974 Expanded Program on Immunization. The WHO's global strategy was to achieve 80–90% Universal Childhood Immunization with a wide range of vaccines through all national systems in all countries throughout the world.[88] Other international vaccination endeavors included the Children's Vaccine Initiative launched in New York City in 1990. This program added to the vaccination pressure aimed at all children in the hardest-to-reach and poorest places of the world.[89]

Diseases of priority established, vaccine schedule in westernized countries expands and includes Hib

In 1985, the US government had established disease priorities. The IOM had proposed a ranking system to determine the ongoing "diseases of importance"[90] based on the following: the expected health benefits to be achieved by reducing morbidity and mortality to the specific disease and the anticipated net savings of health care resources. This model was applied to fourteen diseases in the United States resulting in a top five: hepatitis B, respiratory syncytial virus (RSV), *Haemophilus influenzae* type b (Hib), influenza, and *Herpesvirus varicellae* (for "high-risk" individuals). This government study concluded that the creation of a Hib vaccine was a high-priority need—giving direction for innovation to pharmaceutical companies.

When this decision was made, the novel conjugate Hib specifically formulated for infants was already in development.[91] Hib is a bacterium that can cause meningitis, an inflammation of the membranes covering the spinal cord and brain. While it had been successfully treated in the past with antibiotics, the bacterium was becoming resistant to this treatment. According to research, the pathogen was responsible for the majority of systemic infections in children in 1981.[92] An estimated 0.5% of all US children developed a Hib infection,[93] and 5%[94] of these (0.025% of all children) would die from complications of the disease. However, US national mortality rates for Hib were already naturally decreasing between 1980 and 1987, an average of 8.5% each year. Between 1988 and 1991, mortality to the disease decreased by 48%.[95] This rapid drop was credited to the introduction of Hib vaccines.

The PRP (haemophilus b polysaccharide, polyribosylribitol phosphate) vaccine for Hib was licensed in April 1985 in the United States for children over two years of age. While it was not without concerns during clinical trials,[96] PRP was used by Praxis in the manufacture of b Capsa 1, by Lederle in HibImmune and by Connaught in HibVAX. However, responsiveness to PRP was age dependent. It was ineffective in children under eighteen months of age and had variable effects in two-year-olds.[97] A solution to this was already in development—the conjugate vaccine.

The bacteria for which conjugated vaccines are designed have an important structural feature in common. They are surrounded by a thick and slippery capsule. The Hib capsule is made of carbohydrate and provides a target for attack by the immune system. Antibodies to the carbohydrate can bind to the capsule and enable the white blood cells to destroy the bacterium.

However, the immune systems of children under two years of age do not respond to carbohydrate antigens. Because of this fact, a vaccine was created that linked the carbohydrate antigen with a toxic carrier protein to which an infant's system could respond.[98] The conjugate vaccine for Hib consisted of a

SEVERE LIFE THREATENING ALLERGIES
SURVEY RESULTS
September 2000

NUMBER OF SCHOOLS RESPONDING TO THE SURVEY:26

NUMBER OF STUDENTS WITH LIFE THREATENING ALLERGIES

GRADE	BEE	DAIRY	NUTS	LATE X	SEAFOOD	OTHER	TOTAL
JK	2		2			Chocolate	5
SK	3		12	2		Metal	18
1	2		6			Soya	9
2	1	1	2			Unknown	5
3	2	1	2	1			6
4	3		2				5
5	4		1		1		6
6	2		2			Unknown	5
7	3	1	4	1	2		11
8	3	1	1	1			6
Grades Not Specific	5		6				8
Teachers				2		Perfume Unknown	4
Number of Schools	15	4	18	2	3	5	
TOTAL	30	4	40	7	3	7	90 (4 of these are teachers)

Note: The survey did not request for all allergies to be recorded, only those considered severe, life threatening.
Note: Six students have a combination of allergies (e.g.. Dairy and nuts). These students were only counted under one category.

Figure 1: *Severe Life Threatening Allergies, Survey Results* (Sept. 2000).
A principal at a southern Ontario, Canada, school board was curious about the rising phenomenon of allergy. The principal polled other elementary school principals in the board to determine the number of children with life threatening allergies. Results of this confidential survey revealed that in the 26 responding schools there were 84 children with anaphylaxis. 40 children born between 1987 and 1996 were allergic to nuts and another 30 were allergic to bee stings.
Image credit: Rita Hoffman.

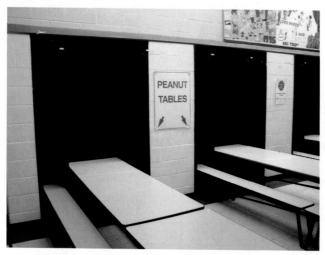

Figure 2: Peanut-designated tables in an elementary school lunchroom, Toronto, Ontario, 2009. At some Toronto schools in 2009, any child with a food item that "may contain" peanut or nut was segregated at the Peanut Table. Peanut allergy had become the new normal and peanut products a politically incorrect choice. By 2014, however, this method of managing the allergy at this particular school was replaced by a complete ban on peanuts and nuts.
Photo credit: Heather Fraser

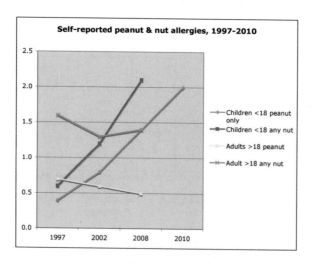

Figure 3: In 2010, researchers observed a steady rise in US self-reported peanut and nut allergies in children under 18 while the adult prevalence remained relatively steady. Anecdotally, this trend has continued and deepened in the US. Chart based on data from S.H. Sicherer, et al., "US prevalence of self-reported peanut, tree nut, and sesame allergy: 11-year follow up," *J Allergy Clin Immunol.*, 125, 6 (June, 2010): 1322-1326; and R.S. Gupta, et al, "Understanding the prevalence of childhood food allergy in the United States," *Pediatrics* (July, 2011).

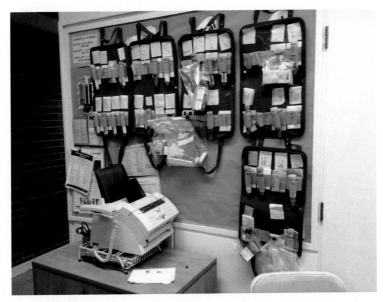

Figure 4: The Allergy Wall is a common sight in elementary schools today. At this Toronto school of about 600 elementary students (aged 4 to 11) approximately 80 children (13%) have been diagnosed with anaphylaxis and prescribed epipens and other medications. This particular Wall has photos, descriptions and medications for juniors only, up to age 6 or 7. These children are too young yet to carry their meds with them. Senior students carry their epis in fanny packs or knapsacks. Photo credit: Heather Fraser, 2015.

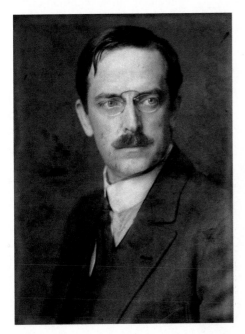

Figure 5: Clemens von Pirquet (1874–1929) was a practicing doctor of medicine at the Children's Clinic in Vienna when he observed the hypersensitive reactions many children were having to vaccination. To describe this reaction in the children, he coined the term allergy (altered reactivity) in 1906. Photo: public domain.

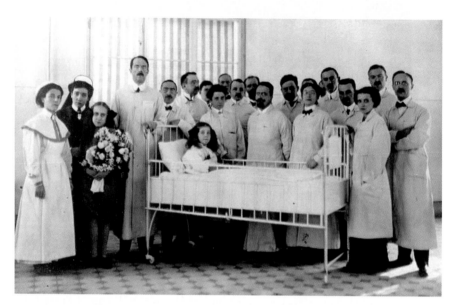

Figure 6: Von Pirquet at the Vienna Children's Hospital c. 1900.
Photo: public domain.

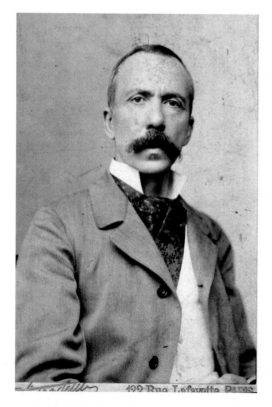

Figure 7: Charles Richet (1850-1935) won the Nobel Prize in Medicine "in recognition of his work on anaphylaxis" in 1913. He coined the term anaphylaxis (against protection) in 1901 following failed experiments to vaccinate dogs to the poison of the Portugese man o' war (physalia).
Photo: public domain.

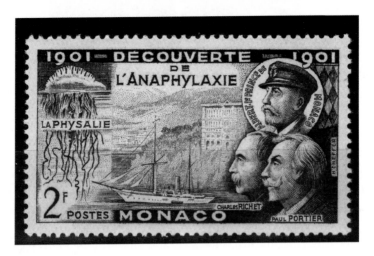

Figure 8: Stamp commemorating in 1953 the "discovery" of anaphylaxis by Richet and colleagues that included the Prince of Monaco during failed attempts to vaccinate dogs to the poison of the Physalia physalis. The experiments were conducted in 1901 on board a ship owned by the Prince. Photo: public domain.

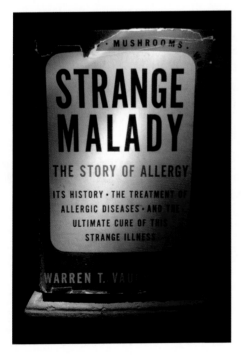

Figure 9: Allergist Warren Vaughan (1893-1944) wrote *Strange Malady* (1941) to help explain allergy to the thinking layperson. In his book, he lists many foods to which people were commonly allergic in 1941 such as milk, egg, strawberry, wheat, etc. Peanuts, however, were of no concern at all – in fact he mentions crushed peanuts as a pleasant food topping only. Allergy to peanut appears in medical literature as a minor concern related to pharmaceuticals containing peanut oil starting in 1948. Allergy to peanut appears sporadically but increasingly in medical literature until the 1990s, at which time mention of peanut allergy in the literature increases dramatically. Photo: Heather Fraser, 2015.

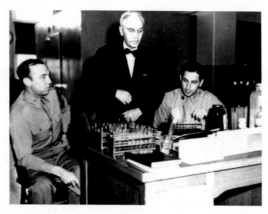

Figure 10: Penicillin pioneer Alexander Fleming (1881-1955) stands next to US Army Medical Corps Captain Monroe Romansky (1911-2006) (right side of photo) at the Walter Reed Army Medical Center. Romansky had discovered a method of prolonging the action of injected penicillin in 1945 by mixing it with beeswax and peanut oil. POB (penicillin in oil beeswax), also known as the Romansky formula, doubled penicillin blood levels but not without some undesirable allergic reactions. It should be noted that the common inclusion of refined peanut oil in pharmaceuticals at this time did not result in epidemic allergy to this food. The epidemic began suddenly starting in the late 1980s through early 1990s.
Photo: public domain.

Figure 11: When a link was made between vaccination and autism, the US government, vaccine makers and the media attempted to squash it. The manner in which this issue was addressed offers a glimpse into the future of research into causes of peanut allergy. The *Green Vaccine Campaign* was launched by Generation Rescue, a non-profit organization in California dedicated to the support of autistic children and their families.
Green Vaccine Campaign ad © Generation Rescue 2010 reproduced with permission
http://www.generationrescue.org

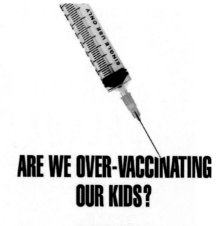

ARE WE OVER-VACCINATING OUR KIDS?

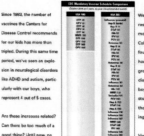

Since 1983, the number of vaccines the Centers for Disease Control recommends for our kids has more than tripled. During this same time period, we've seen an explosion in neurological disorders like ADHD and autism, particularly with our boys, who represent 4 out of 5 cases.

Are these increases related? Can there be too much of a good thing? Until now, no one could know for sure, because no study had ever been done to compare the rate of neurological disorders between

We commissioned a market research firm to survey more than 17,000 children in California and Oregon. We found that vaccinated boys had more than a 2.5 times greater rate of neurological disorders than unvaccinated boys. We believe a national study must be done to further explore these disturbing results.

Visit our site and read the results of our survey, as well as find helpful information on how to vaccinate your child more safely. **Learn more at**

```
Report#    1034
AEFI reports following Penta administered 1994-1995 for age group 6mts-2yrs


Reference Number:        Date received:         Year vaccinated:
V9591779                 1995-07-05             1995


Age group:               Outcome:               Medical attention received:
Toddler                  Fully recovered


Number of vaccine given:
3


Vaccine                  Number in series
Act-Hib                  4
DTP-IPV                  4


                                    _____Onset_____      _____Duration___
WHOART PREF                         Days Hours Mins      Days Hours Mins

General Description:
HIVES ON ARM,TRUNK,LEGS.BEDTIME HIVES JOINED TOGETHER SOLID RASH. CONTINUE WITH IMMUN. SCHEUDLE.CONSUL
T A PEDIATRIC ALLERGIST.



Report#    1098
AEFI reports following Penta administered 1994-1995 for age group 6mts-2yrs


Reference Number:        Date received:         Year vaccinated:
V9790654                 1997-08-07             1994


Age group:               Outcome:               Medical attention received:
Toddler                  Fully recovered        Non-urgent visit


Number of vaccine given:
2


Vaccine                  Number in series
Act-Hib                  1
DTP-IPV                  1


                                    _____Onset_____      _____Duration___
WHOART PREF                         Days Hours Mins      Days Hours Mins
NERVOUSNESS                          .    .     .          .    .     .

General Description:
TYLENOL GIVEN Q4H, BATHS, HYPER-VENTILATING FLUSED 15MIN.CRANKY.RED/PUFFY 4',HARD.LIMP,WHEEZY,HYPER-VE
NTIILATG REFER TO ALLERGIST BEFORE CONTINUING INTO IMMUNIZATON.



Report#    1103
AEFI reports following Penta administered 1994-1995 for age group 6mts-2yrs


Reference Number:        Date received:         Year vaccinated:
V9891432                 1998-06-09             1995


Age group:               Outcome:               Medical attention received:
Toddler                  Fully recovered


Number of vaccine given:
2


Vaccine                  Number in series
Act-Hib                  4
DTP-IPV                  4


                                    _____Onset_____      _____Duration___
WHOART PREF                         Days Hours Mins      Days Hours Mins
HYPOTONIA                           2    .     .          .    .     .
PALLOR                              2    .     .          .    .     .

General Description:
PALLOR & LIMPNESS-NO MENTION OF LEVEL OF CONSCIOUSNESS.,ER DR.DX SHOCK,ALLERGY CONSULT
```

```
Report#    1137
AEFI reports following Penta administered 1994-1995 for age group 6mts-2yrs


Reference Number:        Date received:            Year vaccinated:
V9591662                 1995-07-05                1994


Age group:               Outcome:                  Medical attention received:
Infant                   Fully recovered


Number of vaccine given:
2


Vaccine                  Number in series
Act-Hib                  3
DTP-IPV                  3


                                                 _____Onset_____      _____Duration___
WHOART PREF                                      Days Hours Mins      Days Hours Mins

General Description:
RED,FLAT RASH-GENERALIZED.FAMILY HISTORY OF ALLERGIES. RED,FLAT RASH TO ABDOMEN,CHEST/BACK.SPREAD TO A
RMS,LEGS,EARS. ALLERGIES OF OLDER SIBLING:DOGS,HORSES,SMOKE,PEDIAZOLE.
```

Figures 12-15: There were over 11,000 AEFI (Adverse Events Following Immunization) reports made by doctors to the Public Health Agency of Canada regarding immunization of children under 2 with a Canadian vaccine known as PENTA. Many of the reported reactions over the 3 years this vaccine was routinely administered included allergic reactions and some shock. There were 15 deaths among the reports. There was no apparent follow up on these children to determine short or long term outcomes. PENTA was unlicensed.

Images: reports obtained through Freedom of Information Act from PHAC, 2014.

toxic carrier protein (tetanus or diphtheria toxoids) that was covalently bound to some aspect of the bacterium (i.e., its membrane proteins): a chemical process bonded these two molecules covalently.

The first protein-conjugated Hib vaccine using a protein-carrier diphtheria toxoid (polyribosylribitol-diphtheria toxoid PRP-D) was branded as ProHibit by Connaught. It was licensed on December 22, 1987, for children eighteen months and older. It was relicensed in December 1989 for fifteen-month-old children.

The FDA licensed this vaccine based on a Finnish trial in which thirty thousand children were injected with the PRP-D. It showed 83% effectiveness, but twenty children suffered serious adverse reactions. Another study challenged the efficacy of the PRP-D stating it actually made babies more susceptible to invasive Hib in the window shortly after injection and up to three weeks following administration.[99] The vaccine appeared to depress the immune system.

Other licensed variations of the same conjugate concept quickly flooded the market. As they did, the age limit for their administration quickly dropped for most brands from two years to two months of age:

- December 20, 1989, conjugated Hib vaccine PedvaxHIB by Merck was licensed using PRP-OMP OMP (PRP conjugated with outer membrane protein of Neisseria meningitides) for routine vaccination at fifteen months of age. On December 13, 1990, this brand was relicensed for two-month-old children.
- October 4, 1990, the first of a series of Hib vaccines for two-month-old children appeared, Hib-TITER by Lederie-Praxis. The vaccine used HbOC, a Hib oligosaccharide bonded to a diphtheria toxoid.
- PRP-CRM, another conjugate formulation using protein CRM197, a mutant diphtheria protein. It had been previously licensed for eighteen month olds (December 22, 1988), fifteen month olds (December 1989), and finally licensed for two-month-old children in 1990.
- March 30, 1993, PRP-T by Pasteur Merieux-Connaught Vaccins in ActHIB used a tetanus toxoid as a protein carrier licensed for use on two-month-old children.[100]

In four years, five Hib vaccines were licensed to different companies. These vaccines were marketed, sold to governments, and administered to consumers under the age of two. These vaccines differed in the molecular size of the Hib polysaccharide, the toxic protein used as the carrier, and the methods used to link the polysaccharide to the protein. Thus, according to the IOM in 1994, it is "plausible that variations in the type or frequency of adverse effects may occur because of the differences in the polysaccharide or protein components of the vaccines."[101]

An additional challenge existed in that the Hib vaccine was to be administered at the same time as DPT and polio (OPV). ActHIB, by design, had to be reconstituted by and therefore administered with the combination diphtheria and tetanus toxoids and a whole cell pertussis vaccine.[102] The vaccines were combined for convenience. One shot saved time for parents and reduced the child's discomfort.[103] Doctors blended these vaccines together, literally drawing them into the same syringe from different vials and then injecting this mixture into the infant.

Before the FDA licensed this blend, however, a study was conducted on a group of approximately five thousand Navajo children between July 1988 and August 1990. One report showed efficacy of 90% for PRP-outer membrane protein vaccine (PRP-OMP) in Navajo infants when given at two and four months of age and 100 percent after three doses of oligosaccharide conjugate Hib (HbOC) vaccine given at two, four, and six months of age.[104]

Another nongovernment report described the results very differently. Half of the Navajo babies were vaccinated with five vaccines at once—Hib PRP-OMP, DPT, and OPV—and the other half given a placebo with DPT and OPV. Two doses were given within a follow-up time of about 270 days. What followed was an outbreak of Hib within both groups in 1990. Twenty-three cases were reported. Surprisingly, twenty-two of these infections were in the placebo group. Other infections were reported in both groups and sixteen deaths, according to the nongovernment report.[105]

By 1991, more than seventeen million doses of Hib vaccine were sold in the United States alone. It was a revenue-generating "blockbuster product" according to a 1998 WHO publication.[106] Whether or not there was a general consensus in the medical community regarding the need for extensive use of this vaccine, it seemed that its application had led to a general decline in prevalence of this form of infection in children under five.[107] The human cost of building this immunity, however, was not widely discussed.

With speed and efficiency, the US pediatric vaccination strategy intensified. In 1992, additional doses of combination vaccines were included in the schedule.[108] Between 1993 and 1995, the Clinton administration's Childhood

Immunization Initiative provided federal funds for service, delivery, and immunization programs that peaked at $261 million in state and local awards in 1995. The government's 1994 National Vaccine Plan[109] aimed at 90% coverage of all infants. To that end, the Vaccines for Children Program was adopted as an amendment to Medicaid (1994) providing about $500 million in federal funds for vaccine purchase and delivery. Vaccination also became a requirement before entry to many preschools and day cares.

By 1997–98, childhood vaccination coverage rates reached record highs.[110] The pharmaceutical industry had estimated gross sales of $100 billion in the mid-1980s.[111] By 2008, it was an estimated $500 billion with the market shared by a small number of companies.

Other Westernized countries adopted a schedule similar to that of the United States as recommended by the World Health Organization (six, ten, and fourteen weeks). In Australia, PRP-D, ProHIBIT was licensed in 1992 for infants eighteen months of age. By 1993, HBOC (HibTITER), PRP-T (Act-HIB), and PRP-OMP (PedvaxHIB) were licensed for routine vaccination of infants starting at two months.[112]

In Canada, starting in 1987, a similar progression was made through the Hib vaccines—HbOC (HibTITER), PRP-OMP (PedVaxHIB), PRP-T (tetanus toxoid, ActHIB), and PRP-D (diphtheria toxoid, ProHIBIT) in conjunction with MMR, DPT, and polio at this time. It is important to note that vaccination is not mandatory in Canada and the Ontario Immunization of School Pupils Act was amended to include exemptions in 1984 following protests from the Committee against Compulsory Vaccination. This meant that parents could obtain vaccination exemptions for medical or ethical reasons, but few did so. Vaccination rates in Canada according to WHO data were between 90% and 96% in 1993 and remained high.

The United Kingdom also adopted the WHO vaccination policies and introduced Hib conjugate to the pediatric schedule in 1992.[113] Like the Canadian statistics, the United Kingdom rates in 1990 were 89% to 90% vaccination coverage and remained above 90% through the 1990s.

A suddenly competitive vaccine market spawns the Canadian PENTA, an unlicensed 5 in 1

In 1993, DPT and Hib were included in the first licensed four-vaccines-in-one needle. The first was Tetramune by Lederle. This was followed by OmniHIB from Pasteur Merieux Vaccins. In 1994, five vaccines were packaged into a single needle. The first was a Canadian-made vaccine called PENTA (DPT-Polio-Hib PRP-T) by Connaught (North American arm of Institut Merieux of France later bought by Aventis).[114] PENTA consisted of two separately licensed vaccines: a powdered lyophilized Act-HIB that was reconstituted in a liquid DPT-Polio adsorbed. This combination marketed as PENTA did not receive a drug identification number (DIN) from Health Canada. Nor did it receive approval through a process called notice of compliance (NOC). Rather, in January 1994, the Bureau of Biologics approved through a NOC amendment to the Canadian license for Act-HIB that permitted reconstitution of the Act-HIB with Connaught's DPT Polio Adsorbed vaccine. This product had neither license nor NOC nor product monograph when it was administered to Canadian children starting in 1994. Prior to the release of PENTA there had been one published study on safety or efficacy. In fact, government health officials expressed concern regarding their own ignorance of the safety of this vaccine: ". . . there is insufficient information regarding the lot-to-lot variability in immunogenicity or reactogenicity of PRP-T when given in combination with either DPT or DPT-IPV."[115]

Immediately, reports of adverse reactions to the combination began to pour into Health Canada. In less than three years, there were more than eleven thousand "adverse events following immunization" (AEFI) reports—and reports of this nature are typically 10% of what actually occur. In 2004, a Canadian Department of Pediatrics information sheet stated baldly, "Significant side effects were observed after PENTA vaccination, commonly blamed on the whole cell pertussis component. PENTA was also only about 60–80% effective against pertussis."[116] These side effects included meningoencephalomyelitis (brain inflammation), convulsions, anorexia, infections, anaphylaxis, inconsolable screaming, and death according to Health Canada records. Such was the speed at which this five-in-one combination vaccine was delivered to market. There were no follow-up studies published or made available on these injured children. Ensuing long term damage that anecdotally included both autism and food anaphylaxis was not investigated by Health Canada.

According to the CDC, combination vaccines reduced the number of injections, improved vaccination timeliness and coverage, and reduced shipping and storage costs. Disadvantages were the potential for increased adverse events, extra doses of antigen needed to achieve required antibody levels, and reduced

effectiveness for certain ages.[117] Doctors admitted that unforeseeable incompat-
ibilities when different antigens and chemicals were combined into one vaccine
were distinct concerns.[118]

Starting at two months of age, infants were being administered vaccines
that had been hastily produced and mixed with other vaccines without the benefit of longitudinal studies.[119] The unprecedented schedule had been shaped by
political and economic imperatives and made smooth by legal reforms that
relieved pharmaceutical companies of any serious liability if something went
wrong. It was a perfect storm of international programs and goals that would
have negative implications for certain children and their unwary parents.

The new Vitamin K1 injection, further expanding the schedule

At the same time starting in the mid-1980s, it seemed to go without notice that
the vitamin K1 prophylaxis became routine for newborns in the United States
and many Western countries. Use of the vitamin K as of 2002 was not consistent
in China, by contrast.[120] The purpose of this prophylactic injection was to help
prevent hemorrhagic disease of the newborn (HDN) also known as vitamin
K–deficiency bleeding (VKDB) (*K* for *koagulation*).

Starting in the 1950s and '60s, Western countries, including the United
Kingdom and the United States (AAP, 1961), began dosing newborn infants
with an oral vitamin K1 formula. One brand of the oral vitamin K prophylaxis
was called Synkavite (Roche).

Safety concerns, however, soon arose over the effect of the oral dose
suspected of causing side effects, including hemolysis (destruction of red blood
cells). This problem was addressed by the introduction of an injected vitamin K1
(phytomenadione) that appeared to reduce the prevalence of hemolysis. Routine
use of this product did not begin until the mid-1980s following several reported
cases of HDN in Britain.

Two common brands of the injectable phytomenadione (K1) were Konakion
by Roche and Aquamephyton by Merck. Both products administered to
newborns contained a synthetic petrochemical derived from 2-methyl 1, 4-nap-
tha-quinone in a polyethoxylated castor seed oil base. In studies Konakion was
shown to induce anaphylaxis and was linked to a rise in leukemia in children.[121]
Konakion MM that replaced Konakion in 2006 was made with lecithin E322
derived from soybean and egg.

Little is known about the fate of the ingredients from the injected vitamin K and how well the ingredients are metabolized. The vitamin K1 prophylaxis, which often contains legume proteins, remains as a depot[122] in the leg of every infant starting moments after birth. This depot is held by the child's body for over two months during which time it slowly releases the ingredients that include refined legume proteins. Significantly, this process overlaps with the child's vaccinations at two months of age.

Antibodies to castor seed, while not a true legume, binds to proteins of other oilseed plants such as peanut and soy—which are legumes. A 1987 study in *Plant Physiology* proved that antibody to the castor seed glyoxysomal lipase (62 kDa) also binds to a 62 kDa protein in extracts from peanut.[123]

There was potential that any resulting IgE to castor seed or soybean proteins could cross-sensitize a child to similar dietary proteins such as peanut and nuts. Adding some weight to this potential is the presence of aluminum in some of the vitamin K brands.[124]Aluminum is a known IgE-stimulating adjuvant; 4% of injected aluminum remains indefinitely in the body.

Most peanut-allergic patients also have IgE antibodies against other legume proteins, including soybean. However, "fewer than 15% of such patients react to other members of the legume family."[125] As suggested in the broken-skin hypothesis, a soy sensitization can lead to peanut sensitization through subsequent environmental exposure with reactivity only to the peanut (or to both).

The epidemic of severe food allergy in children arrives

Coincidental with this period of expanding pediatric injections in Western countries was the accelerated prevalence of peanut and other food allergies in children. Unseen by the public, hospital ER records in Australia, the United Kingdom, and the United States documented the upward momentum of food anaphylaxis admissions for children under five. In the United States, ER records showed a steady and rapid increase in anaphylaxis discharges between 1992 and 1994 from 467 per 100,000 to 671. This number jumped to 876 in 1995.[126] In three years between 1992 and 1995, the numbers had nearly doubled. A 1991 US study determined that 90% of all food allergy fatalities were due to ingestion of peanut/tree nuts.[127] The Isle of Wight studies revealed a dramatic doubling of peanut allergy in preschool children in just four years rising from 0.5% in 1994 to 1.1% in 1998.

The same phenomenon occurred in the United States. In 1997, 0.4% of American children under eighteen were allergic to peanuts. By 2002, this number had doubled to 0.8%, and by 2008 the number reached 1.4%. Between 1997 and 2002, the peanut-allergic pediatric population in the United States grew by an average of 58,000 children a year.[128] Between 2002 and 2008, this average annual increase appeared to double.[129] By 2012, as many as 2.3% of Canadian children under 18 and 2% to 3% of children in the US, the UK and AU were allergic to peanut (see Appendix). As children sensitized in the first wave of the peanut allergy epidemic grew into adulthood, the statistic of adults with the allergy began to increase. In 2008, an estimated 1% of the US population was allergic to this one food, about 3 million people. Four years later by 2012, that number jumped to an estimated 4 million living with a life threatening allergy to peanuts. The only word that fits this phenomenon is 'epidemic' and it unfolded in plain sight.

Part 3

PEANUT ALLERGY AT THE CROSSOVER POINT

Chapter 6

—◦◦◦—

ABSORBING THE COSTS

INGREDIENTS: ALUMINUM, FOOD PROTEINS, AND MORE

Vaccination was the elephant in the room. Researchers glanced at it, knew it was there, but were reluctant to get too close. Only a handful of doctors through the late 1990s looked directly at pediatric injections and asked whether a reduction of common childhood diseases through a policy of mass vaccination (and other injections) was worth the price of a higher prevalence of allergy and other adverse outcomes.[1]

Vaccines are a complex blend of antigens, stabilizers, adjuvants, preservatives, antibacterials, antifungals, suspending fluids, gels, and more. While manufacturers, government, and doctors are not obliged to reveal the precise ingredients of vaccines, the CDC offered a limited list.[2] The common childhood vaccine DtaP-IPV/Hib (Pentacel), for example, contains aluminum phosphate, bovine serum albumin, formaldehyde, glutaraldehyde, MRC-5 DNA, and cellular protein, neomycin, polymyxin b sulfate, polysorbate 80, 2-phenoxyethanol. MRC-5 (Medical Research Council 5) is a cell line developed in 1966 from lung tissue taken from a fourteen-week-old fetus aborted for psychiatric reason from a twenty-seven-year-old woman, and more. Bovine serum albumin (BSA) is blood protein from cattle. Neomycin is an antibiotic. Aluminum phosphate is part of an antigen sparing adjuvant.

Adjuvants, as already discussed, stimulate the immune system to respond to just a small amount of antigen. They reduce the cost of a vaccine and increase its efficacy measured in antibodies specific to the disease being addressed. However, they can be dangerous. The choice of adjuvant (or even whether to use one or not) in any vaccine by a maker or government reflects a compromise between immune stimulation and invariable side effects that would be produced in a percentage of consumers. One of the invariable and guaranteed side effects engendered by vaccine ingredients is the production of IgE antibodies.[3] The more effective a vaccine is, the greater the risks of allergies and other adverse effects.[4]

The question about vaccination has never been whether there would be damage but rather how much and what kind in relation to the established vaccination goals. Risk management for the five remaining vaccine manufacturers in the United States was an ongoing concern as the millenium approached. While the FDA had statutory responsibility for licensing vaccines, it appeared to lack the resources to fully grasp all safety issues. In 2004, researchers identified the need for an independent safety risk assessment system.[5] The system of post-licensure vaccine assessment was insufficient and hampered by perceived conflicts of interest.

Before 2000, doctors were beginning to admit that there was an uncomfortable unpredictability in combining different vaccine products in the same syringe.[6] Doctors knew that iatrogenic conditions were being caused by vaccinations, and yet, without comparative data on unvaccinated children, officials were not compelled to reduce the pediatric schedule. In fact, it increased. The possibility of multiple vaccinations causing immune dysfunction was reviewed by the Institute of Medicine in 2002. The researchers admitted that they were unable to reach a satisfactory conclusion on the question. The primary obstacle to resolving the question was that they could not find research on an appropriate control group of unvaccinated children.[7] And the IOM had no authority to conduct its own scientific study.

In 2000 at a meeting of American adjuvant experts fatefully dubbed "thimerosal 2,"[8] doctors admitted that they did not know enough about the absorption, distribution, and excretion of an adjuvant's aluminum from the body especially in infants. "Storage" of aluminum salts that can stimulate autoimmunity and allergy was a problem for some children, they agreed.[9] Birth dose of aluminum, followed by regular doses of aluminum were excreted mostly by the kidneys although in a follow-up study, 4% of the aluminum was still present over three years later.[10] One of the meeting's speakers observed that somewhere in virtually every vaccinated child there remains a depot of the metal that the body does not want to release. Aluminum has an affinity for bone, kidney, brain, and muscle.[11] The hugely provocative nature of aluminum in vaccines was an obvious problem to researchers in a 1978 study who observed that it resulted in a prolonged synthesis of specific IgE in animals: "It is hypothesized that the regular application of aluminium compound-containing vaccines on the entire population could be one of the factors leading to the observed increase of allergic diseases."[12]

Another common vaccine ingredient is gelatin. Gelatin is made from collagen derived from bovine (beef) or porcine (pork) hide and bones. It can also be made from tuna skin.[13] Starting in 1994, a rising prevalence of gelatin allergy in children startled doctors. Children were reacting to many foods that contained gelatin such as marshmallows, fruit gums, yogurt, and vitamin capsules.

A rare admission by Japanese doctors confirmed that there was a causal link between the outbreak of gelatin allergy and the gelatin contained in a new diphtheria-tetanus-acellular pertussis vaccine (DTaP).[14] Japanese doctors acknowledged that an outbreak of gelatin allergy in children was indeed caused by pediatric vaccination. In 1994, changes to the vaccination schedule meant that the DTP was replaced by an acellular version containing gelatin, the age at which it was administered to children was dropped from two years to three months, and it was given before the live virus MMR vaccine that also contained gelatin. A significant rise in anaphylactic reactions to the MMR vaccine given to children at two years of age peaked in 1995 and 1996 after which time vaccine makers removed gelatin from the DTaP. In Japan, discontinuation of gelatin in the DTaP, the MMR, and most other vaccines reduced the rising prevalence of anaphylaxis to the MMR vaccine in children.[15] However, gelatin continued to be used in vaccines in the United States and other Western countries. Doctors admitted that these vaccines were also causing allergies to gelatin in children.[16]

It was perhaps more difficult to conceive of peanut allergy in the same light. The idea that hundreds of thousands of children since the late 1980s had been sensitized to peanut or a reasonable corollary to peanut by ingredients in one or more of the routine pediatric injections was an incredible idea. Doctors seemed surprised that peanut had been used as a solubilizing excipient for decades in oral and injected formulations. "Did You Know This Medicine Has Peanut

Butter in It, Doctor?"[17] the title of this 2007 medical journal article highlights the fact that prescribing doctors did not always know that food products were contained in pediatric medicines.

But the real clue is in the sudden rise in severe allergies to peanut, other foods and bee venom following the significant changes to routine pediatric injections. While contaminant proteins in injections have been proven to sensitize children to foods, it is equally possible that the effect of pediatric injections on the integrity or functioning of the GI system has also contributed to the rise of peanut allergy. No meaningful research has been done into the rise of allergy and the impact of the pediatric schedule on the gut—a system responsible for about 70% of immune function.

SLIPPERY LABELS BUT NO SMOKING GUN

As the peanut allergy epidemic grew, doctors and the government expressed concern regarding the allergenicity of refined peanut oil in processed foods and pharmaceuticals. They debated whether or not it should be labeled. Label reading had become something of a pastime for parents of food-allergic children. If any product listed peanut oil as an ingredient, refined or not, those parents would not purchase it. There were negative financial implications related to manufacturing with peanut oil.

At the same time, demand for the refined oil had increased in the manufacture of processed foods due to concerns over consumption of trans fats. Refined, bleached, and deodorized (RBD) peanut oil was used in fried products, baked goods, and as a flavor carrier.[18] It was considered a healthy alternative to other oils.

But the oil had been shown to cause both sensitization and reactions in a small number of people.[19] The most highly refined peanut oils contain trace levels of intact proteins, up to 0.2–2.2 µg/ml.[20] Lower-quality refined peanut oils could contain 3–6 µg/ml of protein. Thus, in 2004, the European Food Safety Authority (EFSA) investigated the safety of the oil and concluded that "fully refined peanut oil and fat" in foodstuffs could indeed cause allergic reactions in peanut-allergic individuals.[21] The EFSA established a guideline that peanut oil must appear on food labels whether the oil is crude or refined.

In contrast, the WHO Codex Alimentarius Committee on Food Labeling in 2000 had expressed similar concerns but did not render a conclusion: refined peanut and soybean oils in foodstuffs did not necessarily need to be labeled.[22] While this too was a guideline only, the fact that it was laid down by a panel of experts from around the world implied that it was reliable information. Laws would be made based on such on-the-fence guidelines.

The US FDA also acknowledged the presence of trace peanut proteins in the refined oil. However, they chose to grant the oil GRAS (generally recognized as safe) status since they believed no reactions had occurred from its consumption.[23] In the United States, it was not and is not mandatory to label refined peanut or soybean oil in foodstuffs.

But what of the peanut oil used in injectable drugs? Where refined peanut or soybean oil appeared as excipients in parenteral drugs used in Europe, the labeling of these products as of 2001 was required on package leaflets. It was expected that manufacturers should warn users that if one was allergic to peanuts, one should not use this medicinal product.[24] These guidelines were produced by the Committee for Medicinal Products for Human Use (CHMP) at the European Medicines Agency (EMEA). The EMEA helps formulate vaccine package insert statements. Again, these were guidelines with an expectation of compliance and not laws. Deviations from the guidelines, according to the agency, may be allowed if justified on a case-by-case basis. However, in the case of refined peanut or soybean oil, an agency representative confirmed that the consequences of ignoring the labeling guidelines could be serious. Allergic reactions to injected peanut oil in sensitive individuals can occur, stated an EMEA representative: "Patients have a right to know this information, and it is also their right to have it presented to them in a clear, simple, and unambiguous manner."[25]

In the United States, labeling the oil in injected drugs remained voluntary. However, the FDA indicated that inactive ingredients that present an increased risk of toxic effects should be noted in the contraindications, warning, or precautions sections of drug labels.[26] In fact, this labeling option for these ingredients in the United States and Canada was supported by law. Trade secrets that include exact ingredients of pharmaceutical products are exempted under freedom of information legislation in the US, Canada and Britain.

The guidelines and the moral obligation to provide a full list of ingredients were in conflict with laws protecting trade secrets. Again, full disclosure of excipients that included adjuvants, food proteins, and potential side effects was not and continued not to be general practice in the United States or Canada. Thus, labeling became a matter of least legal exposure within carefully worded vaccine product monographs. Whether parents were offered and read the monographs or not was another matter. A search for granted vaccine patents will certainly reveal all manner of vegetable oils including peanut as an ingredient, that may or may not be used. But there are scores of patents that never make it to manufacturing. There is, again, no way for a parent to know precisely what is in a vaccine. To be clear, the author has found no evidence that peanut oil is used in any of the vaccines in the pediatric schedule.

HOMOLOGY OF PEANUT AND HAEMOPHILUS INFLUENZAE TYPE B

Further complicating the outcome of routine vaccination was the apparent homology of the proteins of *H. influenzae* b in the Hib vaccine and the proteins of peanut.

Homology simply refers to the similarity in the structure and the weight of protein molecules of different substances. Homology of molecules leads to cross-reactivity. This phenomenon explains why a person allergic to peanut proteins may also react to nuts, even though they are from different plant families. The protein molecules of peanuts and those of tree nuts are homologous.[27]

The success of any vaccine design is in part built around the molecular weight(s) of the antigen. For example, studies indicate that protein conjugates made with low molecular weight dextran (polysaccharide) were more "immunogenic" than those made with dextrans of higher molecular weight.[28] In fact, molecules liable to bind more readily with blood serum are those with low molecular weight. Researchers have pointed to the low weight of drugs that must bind to carrier proteins in the body to elicit sensitization (less than 1,000 Da) whereas high molecular weight molecules (larger than 5,000 Da) can act as complete antigens and bind covalently on their own.[29]

It occurred to some researchers that Hib proteins, bound to their diphtheria or tetanus toxins or free floating and circulating in the blood stream, could result in an allergy to Hib. Once sensitized to these proteins, there would exist the potential for cross-reactivity to foods of homologous molecular weights: foods such as peanut.

The peanut protein Ara h 1 has a molecular weight of between 20 kDa and 63.5 kDa.[30] A similar range exists for proteins of the Hib outer membrane—between 39 kDa[31] and 98 kDa.[32] While there is a potential for cross-reactivity between the Hib and peanut, there were no apparent formal studies on this relationship.

VACCINE ANTIGENS AS AN ADJUVANT IN CREATING PEANUT ALLERGY

A 1959 study that found mice inoculated with a killed pertussis vaccine easily became allergic to grass pollens. In other words, the vaccination created a life-threatening allergy to a substance in the environment.[33] A similar study took place in the late summer of 1973. Mice vaccinated again with a killed pertussis vaccine became sensitized to ragweed pollen that happened to be in the air at the time.[34] Subsequent intravenous injection of the mice with pollen extract resulted in an anaphylactic reaction. And in several peanut-allergy studies, mice were made allergic to peanuts by inhaling or eating the food mixed with a toxic bacterium.[35]

Thus, the antigens and other toxins used in the vaccines, including the Hib vaccine—diphtheria and tetanus—were also causes for concern. These antigens promoted allergies to the environment and foods consumed following vaccination or injection.

TOXICITY OF HIB-DPT IN CREATING ALLERGY

Anaphylaxis to the Hib vaccine itself, including tetanus and diphtheria toxins it contained, was surprisingly common. The natural bias of the infant immune system toward the Th2 response may have increased this allergic potential within an expanding and intense pediatric vaccination schedule.[36] In fact, by 2000, anaphylaxis following vaccination had notably increased. Doctors admitted that this increase had "complicated" what used to be a routine procedure.[37]

Margie Profet elucidated the purpose of allergy in the vaccination event—whether the serum sickness of the early twentieth century, postwar penicillin allergy, or the massive rise in food allergy in children since 1990, the purpose of allergy is to protect the body against acute toxicity.[38]

Already it was well known that toxins from tetanus and diphtheria bacteria in the conjugate Hib vaccine frequently produced high levels of IgE and anaphylaxis in children.[39] Indeed, bacterial toxins were well-known adjuvants. It was possible, again, that these toxins, which adjuvanted the Hib or other ingredients in the combined vaccines, also enhanced the risk of allergic sensitization to foods in the diet or food proteins in the vaccine.

A 1999 study hammered home this potential. It was found that pertussis bacteria had the ability to induce intestinal hypersensitivity and to prolong sensitization to foods in a mouse model. A mouse injected with ovalbumin (egg) showed IgE in jejunal segments that disappeared by fourteen days. However, pertussis toxin with ovalbumin resulted in long-lasting sensitization present eight months after primary immunization. Bacteria when administered with a food protein resulted in long-term sensitization to the food and the antigen and altered intestinal immune function.[40]

In fact, medical literature was replete with examples of "how to" make an animal anaphylactic to foods by injecting it with toxic pathogens and peanut proteins. For example, mice were made anaphylactic to peanut through injections of heat-killed listeria and peanut,[41] a "cocktail" of measles vaccine and peanut,[42] and mycobacteria and peanut.[43]

But when both Hib and its toxic conjugates were combined with a highly stimulating DPT vaccine, the immune response was even more pronounced. The Hib polysaccharide in a combination vaccine with DPT resulted in a more than twentyfold increase in antibody levels over the Hib alone.[44] This overstimulation of the immune system tipped the scales too far in favor of iatrogenic conditions including allergy.

Again the challenge in vaccine research was to gain potency while minimizing toxicity.[45] Many doctors saw toxicity and allergenicity as an acceptable compromise in the use of vaccine adjuvants. This compromise, for some doctors, was an "accepted principle in the search for adjuvants suitable for use in human vaccines because one of their functions is to stimulate antigen presenting cells."[46] Doctors seemed unaware, however, that the risk-benefit ratio had shifted.

The countries in which the peanut allergy first emerged were those that first paired the Hib with the DPT vaccine. In 1997, Hib was not used in Russia, India, China, the Philippines, Romania, Korea, Iran, Singapore, and other countries where peanut allergy was virtually unknown at that time.

Singapore provided a poignant illustration of the impact of Hib-DPT combination when it was first introduced after 2001. In this country where full immunization of children was enforced by fine and imprisonment, Hib was optional, available for a fee. Since Hib was uncommon in Singaporean children, doctors suggested that the universal Hib vaccination program was not needed.[47] And yet in a surprising turn of events, many Singaporean parents had actually chosen and preferred to vaccinate with the convenient and combined acellular-pertussis-inactivated polio-Hib vaccine (DPTa-IPV/Hib).[48]

This combination had been approved for use in Singapore after 2001. At that time, sensitivity through skin prick tests to peanut showed that the allergy existed in Singapore, but there were no reports of actual reactivity.[49] By 2007, a three-year study revealed a "worrying trend" of peanut reactivity in Asian children living in Singapore (identifying with Chinese, Malay, Indian, and Eurasian ethnic groups).[50] Researchers there underscored the importance of examining environmental factors in this development, but lack of exposure to peanuts was not one of them.

And doctors in Africa were puzzled by the high levels of IgE to peanut in children living in Ghana. Children there had received the five-in-one shot containing DPT and Hib starting in 1992. In 2000, the Global Alliance for Vaccines and Immunization (GAVI) set a goal to fully vaccinate children under the age of one by 2010 in that country.[51] The hyporeactivity of the children was explained by the problematic prevalence of helminths. These parasitic worms depressed immune system reactivity. By 2011, however, 2.5% of children were allergic and reacting to peanut.

But reactions to peanut were virtually nonexistent in Indonesia and seemingly rare in western Siberia, Russia.[52] As of 2005, children were not vaccinated for Hib in Russia.[53] It was set to be introduced after 2010. And as of 2010, a probe study for future use of the Hib vaccine was being conducted in Indonesia.[54]

And in India, where peanut allergy was also not reported, doctors did not vaccinate for Hib. However, a proposal to introduce the vaccine in a pentavalent vaccine was made in 2008. Its proponents claimed it had become cost effective to do so.[55] A sharp rise in the prevalence of peanut allergy might then be expected to occur in India and other countries where a combination vaccine includes the Hib vaccine and there are high coverage rates.

THE AUSTRALIAN EXAMPLE

The history of changes to the pediatric schedules in Tasmania and the Australian Capital Territory provided yet another provocative illustration of how and when peanut allergy emerged.

In a 2001 study, none of the 456 Tasmanian children aged seven to eight years reacted to a peanut skin prick test.[56] By 2009, one in ninety children or 1.11%[57] was allergic to peanuts. Changes in the vaccination schedule and the increased rate of children vaccinated in Tasmania correlated to this development.

In 1997, Tasmanian children were the least likely to be vaccinated at 27% of children according to the Australian Bureau of Statistics.[58] Vaccination rates were dramatically low and declining on this island of about five hundred thousand people. In 1998, only 21% of children were vaccinated by their first year.[59]

In 1998, the Australian government established a General Practice Immunization Initiative that intensified the pediatric schedule and national coverage for preschool children, including those in Tasmania. The goal was to have over 90% of the children vaccinated. In 2001, the Australian government implemented their strategy[60] and surpassed their goal by vaccinating 94% of Tasmanian children by age one. Tasmania became the highest vaccinated population in the country.[61] By 2009, 1.11% of Tasmanian children were allergic to peanuts.

In contrast to the sudden growth of the allergy in Tasmanian, peanut allergy in children living in the Australian Capital Territory (ACT)[62] grew steadily. By 1995, 0.5% of ACT children were peanut allergic.[63] By 2001, 0.71% of ACT children were allergic, and by 2009 2% of "school entrant" ACT children were confirmed as peanut allergic.[64] Children living in this national political center were the most likely to be fully immunized at 48% in 1995[65] according to the Australian Bureau of Statistics. Changes to the pediatric schedule of ACT were similar to but made less rapidly than those in the United States and the United Kingdom. The changes to the schedules for ACT and Tasmania were, of course, the same. But again, the primary difference between Tasmanian children and those living in ACT was vast differences in rate of vaccination. Government programs attempted to harmonize this rate in 2001.

THE VITAMIN K1 PROPHYLAXIS

Most peanut-allergic patients also have IgE antibodies against other legume proteins, including soybean and also oil seed proteins such as castor. However, "fewer than 15% of such patients react to other members of the legume family."[66] As suggested in the broken-skin hypothesis, soybean sensitization can lead to peanut sensitization through subsequent environmental exposure to peanut but with reactivity only to the peanut.

As discussed in chapter 5, since the mid-1980s the United States, the United Kingdom, Canada, Australia, and many other Western countries have routinely administered a prophylactic injection of a vitamin K1 to virtually all newborn babies. The use of vitamin K as of 2002 was not consistent in China, by contrast.[67] The purpose of this prophylactic is to help prevent hemorrhagic disease of the newborn (HDN) also known as vitamin K–deficiency bleeding (VKDB) (*K* for *koagulation*). This injection has commonly contained castor seed oil.

The administration of an oral vitamin K1 formula began in many Western countries during the 1950s and '60s. However, there were side effects. This oral dose was suspected of causing hemolysis (destruction of red blood cells). This problem was addressed by the introduction of an intramuscular or subcutaneous vitamin K1 (phytomenadione) injection that appeared to reduce the prevalence of hemolysis. However, routine use of this product did not begin until the mid-1980s following several reported cases of HDN in Britain.

The injectable vitamin K1 (phytomenadione) prophylaxis known as Konakion by Roche also contained Cremophor EL, a polyethoxylated castor oil. Seven hundred twenty-eight million children were injected with Konakion or Konakion MM between 1974–95, 95% with Konakion.[68] Aquamephyton by Merck is a synthetic petrochemical derived from 2-methyl 1,4-naptha-quinone also in a polyethoxylated castor seed oil base. In the studies, Konakion was shown to induce anaphylaxis and was linked to a rise in leukemia.[69] Konakion MM that replaced the ubiquitous Konakion in 2006 was made with lecithin E322 derived from soybean and egg.

While the food products used in these pharmaceuticals were refined to reduce the sensitizing proteins in them, it was and continues to be impossible to remove them all. And it is well known that antibodies to castor seed bind to proteins of other oilseed plants such as peanut and soy. A 1987 study in *Plant Physiology* confirmed that antibody to the castor bean glyoxysomal lipase (62 kDa) also binds to a 62 kDa protein in extracts from peanut.[70]

The injected ingredients of the vitamin K1 shot remain as a depot[71] in the child for an extended period of time. This depot is metabolized gradually, the ingredients released into the body over the course of a few months. Little is known about the fate of the ingredients, but this metabolizing process overlaps with the vaccination schedule. When the child receives his first vaccinations at birth (Hep) and/or at two months of age (DPaT-IPV Hib), the vitamin K ingredients that include seed or legume proteins are still being released.

There was a real potential that resulting IgE to castor or soy could cross-sensitize a child to similar dietary proteins such as peanut and nuts. Adding weight to this potential is the presence of aluminum in some of the vitamin K brands.[72] Aluminum is a well-known IgE stimulating adjuvant, 4% of that injected also remains indefinitely in the body.

IDIOSYNCRASIES: THE ABILITY TO DETOXIFY

But if the schedule of pediatric injections was somehow sensitizing children to peanut or homologous proteins, why were all children not allergic? Why, even in the same family, was one vaccinated child peanut allergic and another one was not?

Allergy is designed to defend against toxins that escape general detoxification. This being true, the potential for allergic sensitization to drugs and the ability to detoxify those drugs are inversely related, suggested Profet.[73] The ability of peanut-allergic children to eliminate toxins, including those from the pediatric injections, would have been challenged at the time they were administered and afterwards.

Bock pointed to four catastrophic changes that have contributed to the rise of allergy as well as asthma, autism, and ADHD: toxins have proliferated, nutrition has deteriorated, vaccinations have increased, and children's abilities to detoxify have dwindled. Methylation and sulfation, two important detoxification processes responsible for removing mercury and other toxins, have been damaged, suggested Bock.[74]

Children with severe allergy exhibit an immune system overload[75] caused by antibiotic overuse, fungal overgrowth, overactivitiy of the Th2 cells, childhood vaccinations and injections, and more. The fungal infection that began in the gut was made worse by poor eating habits and deficiencies in nutrition, probiotics, essential fatty acids, stomach acid, and digestive enzymes. Further challenging the child was maternal health. Fungal infection was passed to unborn children. Birth by cesarean that delayed the introduction of healthy digestive flora would only have exacerbated the condition.

Gender also played an enormous role in who developed the peanut allergy. The allergy appeared more often in boys than girls—the ratio greater than 2:1.[76] A male predominance of peanut and tree nut allergy was reported in children younger than eighteen years—1.7% versus 0.7% males to females.[77]

While there was no clear explanation for this disparity, a parallel phenomenon had occurred in the prevalence of autism where boys were affected more than girls in a 4:1 ratio. This gender gap was as high as 10:1 for Asperger's syndrome. In 1964, Bernard Rimland observed that boys tended to be more vulnerable to "organic damage" than girls whether through hereditary disease, acquired infection, or other conditions.

The rate of autism and peanut allergy in children increased within the same window of time starting around 1990 with a concomitant sex ratio difference. The rate of autism in the United States was believed to be one in one thousand in 1970.[78] In 2009, it was more than one in one hundred children in the United States by 2014 this number was believed to be 1 in 68 children with 1 in 25 boys being affected. Peanut allergy had a small but growing profile prior to 1990. In 2008, an estimated 1.4% of US children were allergic to peanuts. And 2 years later, this number had jumped to 2% (see Appendix).

And so, children with an extant immune overload caused by various deficiencies and impaired detoxification processes responded adversely to the new and intense schedule of injections launched in the late 1980s and early 1990s. It was a final straw. And within this scenario it is possible that all the four A conditions may, in fact, exist to some degree in every child who has reacted adversely to vaccination. For example, the child with food anaphylaxis also has a "touch" of ADHD and struggles with fine motor skills; the child on the autism spectrum has a food intolerance and often anaphylaxis; the child with ADHD has food intolerance and a touch of asthma but only when he gets a cold—in short, although perhaps undetected one of the As may not exist without the presence of the others in a tragically rounded dissonance to a variety of substances inside and outside of the body. The four As are not parallel phenomena but may coexist within an umbrella condition precipitated by vaccination.

Screening children before vaccination would have been a way to reduce risks of injection but was not common practice before the terrific increase in allergies that has occurred. Even with the few questions posed to parents prior to vaccination, no inquiry was made into the child's sulfation and methylation processes, kidney health, mitochondrial function, or whether mother and child had fungal infections.

A vetting process based on idiosyncrasy was antithetical to the aims of mass and routine vaccination. A thorough screening would also challenge the cost effectiveness of vaccination. Vaccination was alleged to save money otherwise lost should working parents have to stay home to care for their sick children. This affected the national economy. And if many children were found to be at high risk of adverse reaction, they would have to be exempted from these injections. How would society manage this scenario?

Conversely, what was the financial cost of peanut allergy to society? Since the parents and allergic children absorbed the damage, there was little or no financial burden on government or society although it challenged the peanut industry—that appeared to fight back with a genetically modified and impossibly "hypoallergenic" peanut or helping fund a study offering an unsteady conclusion that we might need to eat more peanuts to help prevent allergy. Peanut-allergy families coped through avoidance strategies, and school communities modified their behavior to accommodate the growing problem. Alternatively, revenues were being generated through peanut- and other food–allergic children in the United States—almost six million children in 2008 but that number probably being much higher and with a bullet—fueled a burgeoning food allergy industry through the purchase of drugs and free-from foods.

Chapter 7

—∞∞∞—

RATIONALIZATIONS

THE CROSSOVER POINT

In 2014, there was about a one in thirty-three chance that a child, especially a male living in the United States, Canada, the United Kingdom, Australia, and a handful of other Western countries would develop peanut allergy. When asked what was causing this epidemic, doctors deferred to the hygiene hypothesis or simply stated that they did not know.

And yet, medical literature illustrated that the only means by which immediate and mass allergy had ever been created was by injection. With the pairing of the hypodermic needle and vaccine at the close of the nineteenth century, mass anaphylaxis made its explosive entry into the Western world. Serum sickness from this new procedure was the first mass allergic phenomenon in history specifically in children. Epidemic allergy to penicillin reminiscent of the "days of serum sickness" emerged with its global application following World War II. And with this drug allergy came low prevalence of peanut allergy. Penicillin was administered using a peanut oil base in POB and PAM during the 1950s through the '60s. The use of refined peanut oil in drugs and vaccine adjuvants continued through the 1960s coincidental with the slow growth of the allergy until the late 1980s. Around 1990, prevalence of peanut allergy in children exploded. Extensive and sudden changes to childhood injections and coverage rates precipitated this new mass allergy.

But what precise combination of ingredients within these injections was responsible? Was it a cross-sensitizing Hib protein or castor seed oil from the newborn vitamin K1 prophylaxis followed by consumption of peanut, IgE stimulating toxic antigens, or any of these combined with a dose of aluminum salts within the novel five-vaccines-in-one shot? The potency of the new schedule had the power to sensitize a child to what was in the shot, the body or the air at the time of injection. Did the injections cause gut inflammation and permeability then predisoposing children to allergy? Preexisting conditions such as the all-too-common gut fungal infections further complicate the pediatric schedule.

Whatever the precise mix of ingredients—and it might not be the same for every child—there were so few precipitous candidates that could touch just children, only in certain countries and at the same time, that injection was the most obvious suspect. And again, injection was the only mechanism with a history of having created exactly this condition in children en mass starting over one hundred years ago. This sudden acceleration between 1988 and 1994 was the primary clue. One could not argue with ER records, statistics, eyewitness accounts (including the parental refrain "no one had peanut allergy when I was at school"), and cohort studies that all pointed to a specific window of time in which peanut, other food allergies and atopy in children began to increase.

What could have had the power to create this defense against acute toxicity in hundreds of thousands of Western children at the same time in history to the same proteins? Coincidence, peanut oil skin creams, or genetics failed to explain this abrupt phenomenon. And if digestive failure was to blame, what would cause an abrupt increase in this kind of bowel "dysfunction" in children just in these certain countries at the same time? Antibiotic use, herbicides and GMOs erode the integrity of the gut but these could not, again, explain the abruptness with which prevalence of the allergy increased.

Doctors knew that as the number and potency of vaccines increased, so, too, would the risk of side effects that included soaring IgE and atopy.[1] Anaphylaxis immediately following vaccination had finally become an "obstacle" to the routine jab, doctors observed.[2] But any suspicion that peanut allergy was precipitated somehow by vaccination, however, was quickly muffled and trapped within a complex weave of conflicting agendas held by government, medical authorities, pharmaceutical corporations, and the media.

At stake in any hint of culpability were the reputations and incomes of doctors and scientists, the interests and power of medical associations, massive corporate revenues, shareholders interests, the authority of government, and its control over the health of entire populations.[3] It was a rare doctor who stepped outside of this awesome mesh to wonder in print whether multiple vaccines were worth the massive rise in atopy.[4]

There were several rational arguments doctors used for not publicly pursuing the connection between the new expanded schedule imposed on children starting in the late 1980s and the rise in peanut allergy. The first rationalization was that the Vaccine Injury Compensation Program guidelines in the United States made it impossible to prove a causal link between vaccination and a later "onset" of a life-threatening allergy—that is, in the case of peanut allergy, when the toddler begins to eat solids, including peanut butter, months after vaccination. The guidelines only recognized damage that occurred shortly after injection.

Richet himself who wrote that anaphylaxis "perhaps a sorry matter for the individual, is necessary to the species" summarized the second rationalization. "There is something more important than the salvation of the person, and that is integral preservation of the race."[5] The aim of protecting the whole of society from disease through vaccination of children justified the unavoidable casualties. And making this damage public would only dissuade people from giving their children injections.

The third rationalization was economic. Vaccine consumers absorbed the costs of damage. Therefore, it made financial sense on the part of the pharmaceutical companies and governments to ignore the problem—which could not be proven anyway by their rules. The IOM admitted that they were unable to analyze and, therefore, deduce a connection between allergic conditions in children and vaccination because there were no acceptable unvaccinated populations in the United States. There was no control group. Amish communities in which peanut allergy was virtually unknown also discouraged vaccination. However, because these communities were genetically linked their example was inadmissible.

And finally, if sympathetic courts allowed litigation from concerned parents, the government would intercede with legislation to control it as it did in the United States in 1986 with the National Childhood Vaccine Injury Act. This Act provided a no-fault alternative to the tort system in which the US federal government cushioned the relationship between the public and the pharmaceutical companies with new rules and money. The door to possible litigation brought by parents for vaccine injury in their children was firmly closed in the US in 2011 following Bruesewitz v. Wyeth. In this case parents allegations of vaccine injury were denied by the 'vaccine court' and the case went to the Supreme Court. It was deemed that vaccine manufacturers are not liable for vaccine-induced injury or death as long as the vaccines are accompanied by package inserts that outline instructions and risks.

The way individuals experienced risk in society had changed substantially since the days of Jenner or Pasteur. In the early days of vaccination, a social contract of sorts was forged between populations and the medical community that assured people of better odds if they were vaccinated. This may have been proven right or wrong, but the risks were in the open and if you were frightened enough you had the vaccination—mandatory vaccination laws, disease mongering, and scare tactics helped you make a decision, but the risks were evident. As the century unfolded, risks associated with vaccination were delineated for the public by government, politicians, and medical authorities via the mass media. A quick tally of TV news program advertisements reflected the degree to which pharmaceutical companies paid for and influenced the information streaming into every household.

Parents were assuaged by the institutional language of medical officials who explained that "routine immunizations do not increase the risk of babies developing allergic disorders and are safe to give to babies with food allergies, eczema, or asthma".[6] In truth, parents were hard-pressed to know what they were actually doing when they vaccinated their children. Vaccine package inserts did not disclose complete ingredients. As ever, parents, mothers especially, relied on doctors to explain the procedure perhaps not realizing that in the event of an adverse reaction, they and their child would be abandoned by the system they trusted and branded criminals should they stop vaccinating.

The landmark nonfiction horror *A Shot in the Dark* (1991), written by a medical researcher and an angry mother, forced many to think about vaccination from the consumers' perspective. Their book highlighted the degree to which medical authorities and government had shifted responsibility for vaccine damage away from pharmaceutical companies and doctors by placing onus of proof on parents.

Helping parents understand the role of vaccination in the dramatic rise of autism in US children became a cause for parents like celebrity Jenny McCarthy.

McCarthy's nonprofit organization, Generation Rescue, launched a vaccine awareness campaign in 2005. The Green Our Vaccines campaign asked, "Why are we giving our children so many more vaccines so early in life?" US children receive their first injections within moments and hours of birth and a total of thirty-six different vaccines in their first two years. In 1970, when children received about ten vaccines, the rate of autism in the United States was about one in one thousand. By 2014, this number was believed to be 1 in 68 children diagnosed with an autism spectrum disorder.

The epidemic rise of autism parallels that of the peanut allergy in the period of its acceleration and gender ratio differences in children—more boys than girls are affected by both conditions. Many autistic children also have severe food allergies. When a link was made between vaccination and autism, the US government, vaccine makers, and the media attempted to squash it. The manner in which this issue was addressed offers a glimpse into the future of the peanut allergy.

In 2000, a confidential report *Thimerosal VSD Study, Phase I* (2000) from the CDC linked the rise in autism to a mercury based antifungal vaccine ingredient, thimerosal. Eli Lilly and Company, a company founded by Civil War veteran Eli Lilly, developed thimerosal in the 1930s. An emergency meeting held at the Simpsonwood Retreat Center in Georgia was called by the CDC and attended by fifty-two vaccine experts and pharmaceutical company representatives. A transcript of the meeting leaked to the Internet revealed how frightened doctors were by this government revelation. Here was the basis for ruinous class action lawsuits and serious loss of public confidence in vaccination.

While the thimerosal report ultimately was made available, its original supporting data was lost. At the same time, the database of approximately one hundred thousand children on which the report was based was given to a private company beyond the reach of the Freedom of Information Act.

In 2000, the maker of thimerosal, Eli Lilly and Company, was shielded from prosecution by parents of autistic children when House Majority Leader Dick Armey put the "Eli Lilly Protection Act" into the Homeland Security Act.[7] When this act was repealed in 2003, US Senate Majority Leader Bill Frist in 2008 added a provision to an antiterrorism bill that denied compensation to children suffering from vaccine-related brain disorders. In a post-9/11 world, Frist explained, US companies needed protection from cumbersome and costly lawsuits so that they were free to produce vaccines in the event of a bioterrorist attack.[8]

While the government gradually phased out thimerosal from most childhood vaccines by 2014 the goal of increasing vaccines and maintaining high rates of vaccination was paramount. One doctor at the Simpsonwood meeting stated that injecting vaccines containing thimerosal into all children despite acknowledged risks was preferable to not vaccinating at all:

> My mandate as I sit here in this group is to make sure at the end of the day that 100,000,000 are immunized with DPT, Hepatitis B and if possible Hib, this year, next year and for many years to come, and that will have to be with thimerosal containing vaccines unless a miracle occurs and an alternative is found quickly and is tried and found to be safe.[9]

The doctor's urgent hyperbole revealed much about the two-day meeting; there were nineteen million, not one hundred million, children under five years of age in 2000.

The ethylmercury was phased out of pediatric vaccines but not most flu shots that approximately 50% of pregnant women received in 2012-13.[10] With this move by government, the media attempted to close the case on the causative role of vaccination in the autism epidemic.

A *Time* magazine article gave the "truth" about vaccination accusing all parents who questioned it of putting "the rest of us at risk."[11] The simplistic "us-versus-them" fiction boiled the discussion down into an easy-to-understand concept of personal belief versus public health. This tactic successfully drew attention away from the seminal issue of disease management and adverse events to target and ostracize a new fictitious enemy—a minority of concerned parents who believed their children had been damaged by injections.

No longer patients or even medical consumers, the parents who chose not to vaccinate their children were painted as dangerous and criminally minded people. Some determined Americans, however, fought back. In 2009, a media-driven influenza scare led to federally mandated flu shots that trampled constitutional rights. Concerned citizens were forced to sue their government. A preliminary injunction to halt federal mandatory flu vaccinations in the state of New Jersey was issued in August 2009.[12]

The "us-versus-them" dialectic also drew attention away from the money. Vaccination was less about medicine than it was about economics. Pharmaceutical company CEOs must, by law, protect their shareholders first.

If there was damage, they would not and could not admit it unless it was in the best interest of their company. Case in point, one pharmaceutical company CEO quoted in a 2006 article reflected that the problem with most adjuvanted vaccines was that their potency caused allergies. While his company's brand was not as potent as others, it was safer.[13] This unusually frank disclosure that his product caused fewer allergies was used to sell his company's products and enhance shareholder value.

Government mass vaccinates populations to protect the economy. In deciding, for example, which diseases needed to be addressed first through vaccination, the IOM in 1985 applied an economic model that included the anticipated net savings of health care resources. In 2003, the economic burden of influenza in the United States was an estimated $87.1 billion, including direct medical costs and indirect costs to employers and lost productivity.[14]

This cost-effective justification does not work for the Hib vaccine, however. In comparing the treatment costs averted by a theoretical burden of Hib and the cost of the vaccine application, a 2005 article supposed that vaccination would reduce direct disease costs by $18 million and decrease productivity losses by $50 million.[15] WHO publications described the Hib vaccine as a "blockbuster" product.[16] The vaccine market in 1998 was an estimated $5.4 billion and was expected to increase by 12% a year. The revenues generated by sales of the vaccine were enormous compared to the theoretical savings in this instance.

In 2006, the pharmaceutical industry profits increased $8 billion in the six-month period following the start of the new US Medicare drug program on January 1, 2006. Profit in 2006 in just six months for the top 10 makers was $39,780,689,350.[17]

In addition to theoretical cost savings for government and corporate profits, there were concrete cost downloads to consumers. The costs of vaccine damage such as allergy were not built into the government model of disease management because they were absorbed by those affected—children and their parents. These people, in turn, have spawned a new source of revenue for business. The rise in food allergy and intolerance has contributed to an enormous free-from food market. The market for gluten-free, lactose-free, peanut-free, sugar-free, and other free-from foods was an estimated $3.9 billion in 2008.[18]

The massive rise in chronic degenerative conditions in children has made money for investors in pharmaceutical stocks, as well. One market analyst suggested that given the explosion in allergy in children that an "autoimmune index" would be a useful tool for investors. This index would help them choose profitable pharmaceutical stocks relative to the rise in such childhood epidemics as peanut allergy, Crohn's, MS, and diabetes.[19]

Was it more profitable to continue producing allergy than it was to change the schedule of pediatric injections and screen children to prevent the allergy in the first place? If it is, the ensuing damage will be paid for by society in years to come. Society has borrowed on the future. And what of the role of parents in making and supporting the tradition of mass injections including the vitamin K1 prophylaxis and vaccines? Society as a whole must share the responsibility for producing the epidemic.

Shaw opined in the preface to the *Doctor's Dilemma* (1909), "Until there is a practicable alternative to blind trust in the doctor, the truth about the doctor is so terrible that we dare not face it." Yet by 2009, one hundred years after Shaw's vitriol and the first decades of the tradition of mass injections, the balance between fear of disease and the risk of side effects has shifted. Medical consumers, especially parents of the millions of children with autism and anaphylaxis, have or are developing a new appreciation for the risks related to vaccinations.

This change in public tolerance was a red flag to Stanford University School of Medicine Dr. Eugene Robin.[20] This elderly doctor pointed to the shifting of the ratio in the number of cases of a given disease to the complications caused by the vaccine. It was a process he called the crossover point where the complication rate of a vaccine for individuals becomes higher than the adverse effects of the disease.

Robin asked readers, including government and pharmaceutical companies, to consider a scenario in which a highly effective vaccine over time progressively decreases the incidence of the disease. When the percentage of adverse events associated with the vaccine remained constant or even increased as the disease became less threatening, society will have reached the crossover point. At that point, wrote Robin, the wise thing for uncomfortable parents to do would be to refuse vaccination.

Parents of autistic children reached the crossover point in 2000—bands of parents in the United States became organized, well-informed, and militant. These groups include The Thinking Mom's Revolution, Autism One, Generation Rescue, The Canary Party, Health Choice and Autism File Magazine and Autism Media Channel.

Parents of peanut-allergic children, however, were coping. But as the epidemic prevalence of peanut and other life-threatening food allergies in children increased, these parents, too, began to take a stand.

PERSONAL POSTSCRIPT: RED FLAGS

Laws and policies related to routine and mass vaccination highlight the extent to which the state controls the bodies of its citizens. Citizens exposed to the media-filtered spectre of disease are asked to relinquish their right to control the health of their children in routine immunization. This many parents do despite vaccination exemptions and without individual screening in exchange for a promise of protection offered by government in the concept of herd immunity.

Let's have a look at that.

The concept of herd immunity is a mathematical model developed in the early 20th century. The complex math is based on variables of susceptible, infected and immune individuals—the goal is to reduce through vaccination those susceptible in order to suppress transmission of a disease.

The math attempts to project the percentage of a population that would need to be vaccinated to suppress a given disease for a period of time. This model, however, may include unrealistic assumptions: the perfect efficacy of the vaccine, that it is a single vaccine, that the vaccine causes no injuries, diseases don't mutate, the suppression of one strain will not alter or create other strains, vaccines don't shed and spread disease, and that there are few contraindications.

Allergies used to be straightforward contraindications for immunization through the 1960s in England and the former East Germany and even Russia until 1994. Eczema is still a contraindication for small pox vaccination—eczema vaccinatum is potentially fatal. Asthma, rhinitis, eczema, food or environmental allergies used to be red flags.

Contraindications today are listed on vaccine package inserts or government web sites including the CDC. These sources indicate that anaphylaxis to any vaccine or vaccine component means you should not be vaccinated with it again. Further, some flu vaccines may not be suitable for children with asthma or wheezing or if they are allergic to antibiotics, gelatin or eggs. Some children should wait or not get the MMR vaccine if they are allergic to neomycin, have a low platelet count or are unwell. Allergies to certain antibiotics are a significant concern as is allergy to latex depending on the vaccine. Epilepsy or nervous system problems are also a serious concern. Inconsolable screaming and seizures following the DTP shot in particular means this shot may be inappropriate for your child. Another red flag.

With such complex and real variables, the mathematical herd immunity formula can vary significantly from reality. This has clearly been the case for recent measles outbreaks in highly vaccinated populations in Canada and the US. A June 2014 HuffPost article containing an interview with a top vaccinologist Dr. Greg Poland describes the current measles vaccine offered in the MMR shot as inadequate and ineffective. Allergies have become an obstacle to vaccination as have educated people wary of and avoiding the vaccine. Significant MMR-related injuries in Japanese children resulted in a ban on this vaccine in that country. Japan replaced the triple shot with single vaccines; the mumps shot being optional. Is there no herd immunity threshold for mumps?

Parents being asked to accept the concept of herd immunity are looking closer at the fine print.

Each disease in the model of herd immunity has a different projected threshold. And yet, parents are led to believe that coverage rates to achieve herd immunity for all diseases are 90% to 95%. A thinking person might wonder if this high blanket number is a convenience. This same person might point out the inherent conflicts in a liability free mandated consumption of vaccines. Neither doctors nor government nor manufacturer in Canada has to date been held liable for vaccine injury.

These and other concerns are making their way to parents and increasingly into the mainstream media. It was recently revealed in an October 2014 Toronto Star article that Ontario schools have growing exemption rates with one school as high as 40%.

In Canada and the US, the rise in exemption rates has resulted in almost hysterical mass media denigration of parental concerns and a dismissal of those injured. A false narrative of anti-vax and pro-vax camps fueled by social and mainstream media has led to recent changes in exemptions legislation in many states and the erosion of individual rights to govern one's own body.

In the first few months of 2015, in the US, state bills have been proposed that seek to remove vaccination exemptions for children on the grounds of parental personal belief or religion and limit the number of doctors able to give medical exemptions. The net result is a wholesale forced vaccination of children whether they attend public school or are home schooled. The US Dept. of Health and Human Services, National Vaccine Program Office released in Feb., 2015 now has an Adult Immunization Plan with 2020 targets to sway adult beliefs and pressure them to comply through community strategies. There are 13 vaccines including those for flu, tetanus, hepatitis, herpes and HPV for adults 18 and older. It is foreseeable that it will become difficult for adults to attend college or secure employment if they are unvaccinated.[21] This Orwellian potential goes well beyond disease management.

This actual evolving scenario of forced vaccination makes quaint the discussion of vaccine safety.

And yet, I was motivated to write this book by events for which I was unprepared as a new parent when my 13 month old son reacted violently to peanut in 1995. In understanding now the direct causal link between vaccination and allergy and in sharing it here I will somehow have helped parents in future to be better armed in making their vaccination choices, and in fighting to keep those choices.

PENTA VACCINE (1994–97), A CAUTIONARY TALE FOR ALL VACCINE CONSUMERS

Working for the Public Health Agency of Canada is a man whose job it is to redact documents. His work is accomplished by hand with strips of white tape and a keen eye. The redactor reads with deliberation then stretches thick or thin strips over numbers, names, dates, drug reactions and outcomes covering up anything he feels may be indiscreet.

And it would have taken him days to complete the pages I requested in 2011. Under the Canadian Freedom of Information Act I had asked for reports of "adverse events following immunization" (AEFI) from doctors who had injected children with a short-lived 1990s vaccine known as PENTA. But I received only a fraction of what I thought would arrive. Perhaps my request was just too big or too vague. As it was, a swath of 1,274 photocopied reports for one year and for children ages 6 months to 2 years arrived a few months later.

The batch was about 3 inches thick and wrapped in a light brown insulated envelope. The envelope had been damaged in transport and repaired by Canada Post. I cut through fat strips of tape with sober thoughts about what lay inside.

It was a frustrating and upsetting read. Pages yawned with large white spaces where outcomes and descriptions had been removed. The words 'fully recovered' were frequent but as there had been no follow up on these children their recoveries had to be qualified. What had life been like for them the next day, month or year following their shots of PENTA?

And anyone reading the doctor-reported reactions would surely have wondered the same thing. Reactions to PENTA, the first mass administered combination of 5 vaccines in a single needle included: ear infections, furious blinking, anorexia, head banging, asthma attacks, allergic reactions, lethargy, shaking, rapid eye movements, vomiting, somnolence, pallor, "ice cold hands and feet while with fever," hypokinesia (inability or struggle to move), inconsolable screaming and an "abnormal gait following vaccination" where the "child hobbled with valgus deformity of the left leg."

Yet another child experienced "myoclinc seizures with a recommendation to defer immunization." One child "looked doped up" and another was red and swollen from head to toe. There were raised rashes, involuntary muscle contractions, an "oculogyric crisis" (rotating eyeballs) tremors, "abnormal crying," "periods of limpness," and numerous seizures.

Treatments for the children involved a lot of Tylenol, benedryl, 'amox' and other antibiotics. Several kids were hospitalized and in this small batch there were two deaths: following immunization with PENTA one child died from cerebral infarction and the other following autopsy was found to have suffered meningoencephalomyelitis, brain and spinal cord inflammation. (see the AEFI reports for these deaths below).

Since these 1,274 documents represented a fraction of what had been reported over the 3 years PENTA had been used, I made a second request in January 2014 for the balance of the AEFI reports. In February I received a letter from the Public Health Agency of Canada (PHAC) explaining that there would be a three month delay in fulfilling my request. The reason: there were 25,000 pages representing over 11,000 adverse events following immunization with PENTA.

The request: all adverse event reports for all children in Canada who received two vaccines between 1994 and 1997 that comprised PENTA: Act-HIB (DIN 01959034) a powder and DPT Polio Adsorbed (DIN 00605050) a liquid. These two licensed vaccines were mixed to create a third vaccine known as PENTA.

The first vaccine, Act-HIB was originally a liquid containing thimerosal. This infamous mercury-based preservative would have killed the whole cell pertussis component of DPT-polio of PENTA and so it had to be changed: the Act-HIB was dried or lypholized.

Picture it: to make PENTA the doctor or nurse used a syringe to suck up and then squirt the liquid DPT- polio vaccine into the vial of powdered HIB. This vial was then shaken by hand. Shake-shake. Did they hold the vial up to the light, eye-balling the particles as they dissolved? This mixture now known as PENTA was drawn back up into the needle and injected promptly into the child.

And yet . . .

PENTA did not have a license.

The government gave the nod to PENTA by amending the Act-HIB package insert to state that the two licensed vaccines could be mixed. Again, still not licensed but who would know or care?

The manufacturer it seemed was in a terrible hurry to get PENTA to a vaccine market that had just opened up wide, really wide.

As described previously (chapter 5), the US Vaccine Injury Act of 1986 paved the way for new vaccines of greater potency with virtually no liability for manufacturers. It was a de-regulation that set the stage for immediate profits while deferring and downloading all costs of damage. The Act with its compensation program rules all but fully barred vaccine injury lawsuits at the same time as the US IOM came out with a list of 'diseases of priority' for which they wanted vaccines. HIB was at the top of this list despite the fact that prevalence of the disease had been dropping by 8% every year over the 10 years previous to the vaccine's introduction . . . The vaccine was already in development.

There has never been a successful suit brought in Canada against a vaccine maker. And the Canadian pediatric schedule did and does run parallel to that of the US. So, I ask: were Canadian children guinea pigs for this product to be released into the much larger market south of the border?

PENTA was a disaster.

After three years on the market PENTA was removed from use in 1997 for 'significant side effects.' This was something Health Canada strongly suspected before the vaccine was introduced.

In 1994 Health Canada knew that, "there is insufficient information regarding the lot-to-lot variability in immunogenicity or reactogenicity of PRP-T when given in combination with either DPT or DPT-IPV."[22]

In 2004 health officials acknowledged that "Significant side effects were observed after PENTA vaccination, commonly blamed on the whole cell pertussis component. PENTA was also only about 60–80% effective against pertussis."[23]

For the manufacturer of PENTA it wasn't even back to the drawing board—they had used the 3 years that PENTA was still in circulation to create a replacement vaccine. This was smart, seamless business.

For the doctors, it was always business as usual.

For a growing minority of families, the strategy of increasing the potency and number of vaccines starting at birth for all infants that began at this time launched the childhood epidemics of autism, allergy, anaphylaxis and more. And for those who suggest that anecdote is not data—aside from thousands of severely redacted AEFI reports, there is no access to data nor science. This information is shielded from consumers by corporate law.

In Canada there is no meaningful mechanism for complaint, investigation, acknowledgement or even legal recourse never mind justice for vaccine injury. If I'd bought a pack of gum I'd have had more consumer protection. As it was, in accepting the vaccine for my son and trusting the doctor I unwittingly accepted the risks that included death. If I had known this, I would have fled the doctor's office.

My son was first injected with PENTA in Nov. 1994. He reacted badly and the vaccination created allergies to foods including dairy. The dairy allergy was undiagnosed at the time and contributed to ear infections. The doctor prescribed antibiotics for the infections followed by creams for the eczema. His allergies were mounting. The second dose of PENTA to which he again reacted with inconsolable screaming was given in January 1995. More ear infections and more antibiotics followed. His respiratory system became reactive. He was diagnosed with rhinitis and asthma and given scripts for puffers and benedryl. In March 1995, he reacted violently to his third dose of PENTA at 6 months of age. After this shot he screamed inconsolably for hours, writhing in severe pain. I later learned that nurses refer to this reaction as a neuro-scream. It is caused by inflammation within the central nervous system, the brain and spinal cord.

Supported by pharmaceuticals and frequent trips to the ER, my son 'recovered' as the redacted PHAC documents might suggest until age one when he had a severe allergic reaction to peanut. We were handed a lifetime script for EpiPens.

In our progress from healthy patient to dependent medical consumer my son joined a fast growing horde of ill children that emerged as the 1990s unfolded. Society was unaware of the creeping epidemic of anaphylaxis until the kids reached the age of 5 and showed up for kindergarten. Schools across

Canada, AU, the UK, the US scrambled to manage this sudden and mysterious development.

With the help of the PHAC redactor I am still piecing together the short term impact of PENTA. Long term is another matter. PentaProject.net is an information gathering initiative where parents of these children can share their stories.

But I do wonder if it is too late. Should I leave the PENTA tragedy untold, give the redactor a break? No. And for the simple reason that the conditions that gave rise to PENTA still exist. Conditions in which the touted concept of herd immunity was reduced to a footnote in an ongoing story of corporate interest and state apathy or incompetence.

There is still no legal recourse for vaccine injury in Canada, no accountability much less acknowledgement that vaccines are inherently unsafe drugs. In 20 years, nothing has changed for Canadian vaccine consumers except that there are more injuries: in Canada, as many as 13% of children under 18 have life threatening allergies.

Vaccination and allergy/anaphylaxis have an unarguable cause and effect relationship. There are over 100 years of published science and a Nobel Prize that explain how immunity and allergy are two sides of the same coin. Through vaccination one 'side' does not respond without the other and the more potent a vaccine, the greater the risk of creating allergy or anaphylaxis to any substance in or around the body or in the shot at the time of vaccination.

All immunologists and allergists know this to be true. Ask them.

Part 4

FIXING ALLERGY

Chapter 8

THE BUSINESS OF BREATHLESSNESS AND OOZING SKIN

But from indications of such a vague character, really serviceable medicines could not be discovered, most assuredly not in the *materia medica* of the old school, which, as I have elsewhere shewn, is founded mainly on conjecture and false deductions *ab usu in morbis*, mixed up with falsehood and fraud.

Samuel Hahnemann, *Organon of Medicine*, 1833[1]

The medical establishment has become a major threat to health. The disabling impact of professional control over medicine has reached the proportions of an epidemic. *Iatrogenesis*, the name for this new epidemic, comes from *iatros*, the Greek word for "physician," and *genesis*, meaning "origin."

Ivan Illich, *Medical Nemesis: The Expropriation of Health*, 1976[2]

Although today's influenza and cholera epidemics make front-page stories, epidemics used to be far more terrifying before the rise of modern medicine.

Jared Diamond, *Guns, Germs, and Steel*, 1997[3]

Part of it has to do with consumption, there is more exposure to peanuts at susceptible ages . . . But it's more than that. There are factors to do with how we vaccinate our kids very early on in life, how much drugs, antibiotics we give the kids early on in life; all of which tends to predispose more towards allergies.

Dr. P. Vadas, Health on the Line, Discovery Health Network, 2001[4]

Western medicine is rooted in a division of mind and body—for which we might credit philosopher René Descartes (1596–1650) who likened the sick body to a malfunctioning clock: fix it or take out the broken parts and things will go back to normal, maybe. This clock-body metaphor became an ongoing invitation to classify, then re-classify the body and its diseases large and small—the progress of which was marked by *materia medica*, treatises on diseases and their remedies. From the treatises of Pliny and Galen to Floyer, Cullen, Salter, and the plethora of twentieth-century medical journals, the evolution of medical thought drew the gaze of the physician away from the patient and towards conquering his symptoms—for better or worse—that included breathlessness and oozing, eczematous skin.

The nosology of what would be known as allergy and anaphylaxis after 1901 in western medicine was first described by where and how symptoms appeared in the lungs or skin. The word asthma, it is said, came from the Greek *asthmati* used in Homer's poetic saga *The Iliad* (c. 800BC). In the epic poem, during the siege of Troy (1194–1184 BC), Trojan commander Hector collapses with an attack of asthma on the field of battle:

> *ho d'argaleoi echet' asthmati ...haim' emeon*
> He was gripped by difficult asthma, vomiting up blood.[5]

The Greek word *ekzema* for oozing and itchy skin that "boiled out" might date from the mid-eighteenth century. And itchy rash with wheals, labeled *knidosis* in the Hippocratic writings, was further distinguished from other skin issues by the word *urticaria* after the Latin word for nettle in 1769 in the *Synopsia Nosologiae Methodicae* by William Cullen (1710–1790).[6]

Once named, diseases were further delineated by cause, biological process, symptoms, and treatments. This organization of thought and observation in medicine through the Enlightenment, the Industrial Revolution, and the Information Age created what philosopher Michel Foucault (1926-1984) called a medical consciousness. Thus, research and remedy (trial and error) or sheer experimentation where scalable nostrums (Latin for "our remedy") made small fortunes for their makers starting in the nineteenth century, which began the medicalization of the modern society.

In this early period, those afflicted with asthma and eczema bought and consumed nostrums that might be useless, helpful, or even comical—purges and enemas, cold-water baths, cigarettes, combustible powders, and expensive holidays. Other packaged nostrums such as arsenic creams, morphine, opium, and horse-blood salve had serious iatrogenic repercussions.

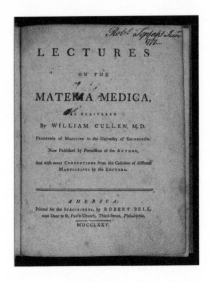

Cullen, *Lectures on the **materia medica*** (Printed for the subscribers, by Robert Bell, next door to St. Paul's Church, Third Street, Philadelphia, 1775).
Credit: Wellcome Library, London

Scottish physician doctor William Cullen (1710–1790) may have been the first to distinguish asthma from general difficulty in breathing or dyspnea in *Edinburgh Practice of Physic, Surgery, and Midwifery*.[7] He identified three manifestations of asthma: spontaneous asthma, exanthematic asthma, and plethoric asthma. For the last, he recommended bleeding and enemas:

> In order to obtain relief in the fit, we must sometimes bleed, unless extreme weakness or old age should forbid, and repeat it according to the degrees of strength and fullness; a purging clyster, with a solution of assafoetida, must be immediately injected; and if the violence of the symptoms should not speedily abate, it will be proper to apply a blistering plaster to the neck or breast.

In his *Treatise of the Materia Medica* (1789), Cullen included opium for relief of "spasmodic asthma" and smoking tobacco for "Its narcotic power applied there often relieves spasmodic asthma; and by its stimulant power it there also sometimes promotes expectoration."

Through the nineteenth century, the causes of asthma were hotly debated. Henry Hyde Salter (1823–71) in his treatise *On Asthma* (1868) defined it as almost "exclusively a nervous disease, the nervous system is the seat of the pathological condition." George Beard (1839–1883), an American neurologist in *American Nervousness*, concluded similarly that asthma was a modern condition brought on by nervous exhaustion.[8]

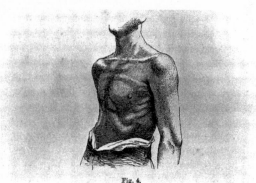

Fig. 4.
From a photograph of an asthmatic, whose disease dated from whooping-cough at three months old.

"Chest of an asthmatic whose disease dated from whooping-cough at three months old."
H.H. Salter, *On Asthma* (London, Churchill,1868) p. 177
Credit: Wellcome Library, London

Yet others believed asthma was the result of affluence like gout, a notion supported by the fashion of hay fever holidays taken by the privileged classes.

Hay-fever tourism was made fashionable by English physician John Bostock (1773–1846). In 1819, Bostock escaped to the coast to avoid summer catarrh that he believed was caused by inhaling "effluvium" from hay:

> With respect to what is termed the exciting cause of the disease, since the attention of the public has been turned to the subject, an idea has very generally prevailed, that it is produced by the effluvium from new hay, and it has hence obtained the popular name of the hay fever.[9]

English physician, homeopath, and hay-fever sufferer Charles Blackley (1820-1900) may have been the first to show that pollens were the likely cause of hay-fever. Experimenting on himself in 1873, he applied pollens to the skin and eyes, in and attempt to "exhaust" the reaction and promote tolerance. Finally, he scratched himself with moistened pollen:

> In a few minutes after the pollen had been applied, the abraded spot began to itch intensely; the parts immediately around the abrasion began to swell.[10]

In America by the late nineteenth century, asthma, rose cold, autumnal catarrh, or hay fever had become "the pride of America's leisure class" and an index of class superiority.[11] Annual migrations to escape effluvium fueled by the wheezing wealthy created an economy of hay-fever resorts. One of the most popular "exempt" locations in the 1870s in the eastern United States were the White Mountains of New Hampshire, according to historian Gregg Mitman. The forests were thought to filter the air "of their noxious elements."[12]

However, those who could not afford the annual escape looked for relief from nostrums—cigarettes, powders, and salves.

In 1802, doctor and asthmatic James Anderson at the Madras Hospital in India had spread the word about smoking datura stramonium; stramonium or thorn apple is in the nightshade family of plants. Its roots and stalks were known for their sedative and antispasmodic properties.

The popularity of stramonium cigarettes like Potter's asthma cigarettes (a preparation of dried belladonna, lobelia, and stramonium) coincided with an increase in other smoking remedies like cannabis, opium, and tobacco—a habit that became widespread through mass production techniques and physician endorsements into the twentieth century.[13] In *On Asthma* (1882), Salter observed that the smoke helped relieve the nervous irritation at the root of spasmodic asthma.

In contrast with Bostock, Blackley, and Salter, physician W. P. Dunbar (1863–1922) in Hamburg reasoned that if asthma was caused by pollen, then everyone should be affected. Instead, Dunbar posited that asthma was caused by

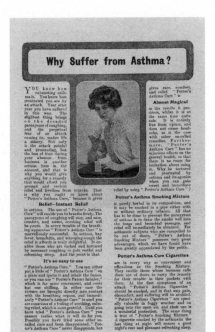

Advertisement for "Potter's Asthma Cure" establishing the effects of asthma on a sufferer and its cure, 1910.

Credit: Wellcome Library, London

a germ and its toxins attached to the pollen. And in the early heroic age of vaccines, the solution for Dunbar was simple—an injected serum.

In 1903, Dunbar created Pollantin, an antitoxin serum made from the sensitized blood of horse or rabbit and pollen. When experiments with the injected serum almost killed his assistant, an unnerved Dunbar reformulated the product as a liquid, salve, pastille, and powder that were applied to the mucous membranes of eyes, mouth, and nose. Dunbar had created a form of passive immunization with Pollantin that resulted in limited relief for a period of time for some users. However, the product was finally pulled from use after a number of users experienced anaphylactic shock.[14]

Equally challenging but less common and certainly unfashionable was the nosology of oozing and cracked eczematous skin. Eczema is not mentioned by Cullen in his *materia medica,* but is included in the homeopathic *materia medica* written in 1810 by Samuel Hahnemann (1755–1843), *The Organon of Medicine.* Hahnemann, a trained physician who discovered and developed homeopathy, recommended dilutions of dulcamara, which under the law of similars or "like cures like" produced "a kind of eczema" in a healthy person. However, he observed that there were several types of eczema with many causes:

> Thus some eczemas are superficially driven off by the external application of cantharides, and other exanthemata by the application of mercurial preparations; but they are not cured in such wise that general health follows, unless these external remedies were capable at the same time of removing the internal morbid state inseparable from the local affection, and unless by their topical application they had affected the whole organism with their curative power.[15]

Allopathic *materia medica* described types of eczema by their lesions, vesicles, and severity. They recommended treatments that appalled Hahnemann:

> To render (through ignorance), if not fatal, at all events incurable, the vast majority (99/100ths) of all diseases, those of a chronic character, by continually weakening and tormenting the debilitated patient, already suffering without that from his disease, and by adding new destructive drug diseases, this distinctly seems to be the unhallowed main business of the old school of medicine (Allopathy)—*and a very easy business it is,* when once one has become familiar

with this pernicious practice and is sufficiently insensible to the stings of conscience![16]

Which appears to have been the case for Charles Darwin (1809–1882) who in his post-*Beagle* years had developed chronic ill health and skin problems that some suggest was the result of an inner conflict between his faith in God and his theory of evolution. Speculation, based on his personal letters, is that Darwin suffered from Crohn's disease and a painful and peeling facial eczema. Between 1859 and 1863, Darwin experienced "attacks" of eczema on his face and head "during which he was hardly recognizable."[17]

Having had the skin condition much of his life, for which he used an arsenic cream, there is further speculation that Darwin may have slowly poisoned himself. In Victorian Britain, arsenic—an odorless and tasteless poison—was used to create a fashionable pigments called Scheele's Green and Paris Green. Used in wallpaper, dress materials, digestive medicines; and whitening complexion wafers and soaps, arsenic was said to have sickened and killed hundreds of people in this period.[18]

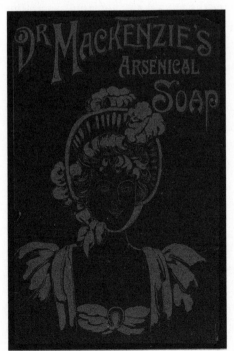

Dr. Mackenzie's Arsenical Soap. 1896. Leaflet or magazine insert advertising bars of toilet soap with "a very small quantity of arsenic" to nourish the skin, whiten the hands, and improve the complexion. It was "guaranteed absolutely harmless". Printed in black on pink paper. The soap was available from S. Harvey, Denman Street, London Bridge.
Credit: Wellcome Library, London
Copyrighted work available under Creative Commons Attribution only licence CC BY 4.0
http://creativecommons.org/licenses/by/4.0/

OF ECTOPLASM, ADRENALINE AND HISTAMINE

At the start of the twentieth century, new understandings about the root causes of asthma, eczema, and urticaria required entirely new labels: anaphylaxis and allergy. The twin relationship of allergy and immunity had emerged from the first use of the hypodermic syringe in mass vaccination (see chapter 4). The triumph of germ theory through vaccination had created the problem of epidemic allergy in children but also an opportunity to analyze, categorize, and then to "fix" it.

As described in chapter 4, French physician Charles Richet (1850–1935) was one of the first to investigate. For his understanding of the pathogenesis and symptoms of anaphylaxis, Richet won the 1913 Nobel Prize in Medicine. But the inquisitive Richet may have chafed at the restrictions of the medical model, with its classification and reclassification of disease and remedy separate from mind and spirit. At the same time, as he was repeatedly unleashing and documenting fatal reactions with the needle on dogs, cats, and horses in the lab, he was investigating paranormal energy that he claimed oozed or squirted from people during a séance. He called this "ectoplasm."[19] A photo of Richet with a medium named Linda taken in 1905 clearly shows a "fluidie thread" of ectoplasm. Attached to this thread released from Linda's head was an ectoplasmic hand. This was "experienced at home in my library" relates Richet.[20]

No doubt, Richet's interest in the paranormal embarrasses allergists today. Truly, ectoplasm is a poor fit for a *materia medica*—it is neither medical nor treatable.

Nevertheless, with the startling discoveries and understanding of allergies and anaphylaxis came the expected merger of science—the new immunochemistry[21]—with the nostrum-monger-turned-pharmaceutical-company. Where the "gaze of the nosographers was a gardener's gaze" in the eighteenth century, observed Foucault, in the nineteenth century it peered sharply into the "quasi-mathematical" chemical operations of the body.[22]

Together, at the beginning of the twentieth century and over the next one hundred years, the scientist and nostrum-pharma companies entered into a lucrative relationship of patented medicines in the new immunochemistry to remedy this "dark side of immunity."[23] From this pairing came: adrenaline, anti-anaphylaxis (desensitization) injections, antihistamines, steroids, inhalers, auto-injectors, novel immunotherapies of skin patches, and capsuless, anti-IgE vaccines, and reprogrammed injected dendritic cells.

PATENTING ALLERGY

In 1847, the American Medical Association deemed it "derogatory to professional character" or even a conflict of interest for a physician to own a patent on a medicine, medical device, or procedure—concerns that disappeared in the latter half of the twentieth century.[24]

Exempt from early AMA ethics was biochemist Jokichi Takamine (1854–1922), funded by Parke-Davis Company in Detroit, who seized the opportunity to patent adrenaline (Latin for "above the kidneys") in 1900 and trademarked the name Adrenalin in 1901. At the same time, other scientists had been attempting to isolate this hormone from the adrenal medulla of animals including Johns Hopkins physician Jacob Abel (1857–1938). Abel had isolated a substance he called epinephrine (Greek for "above the kidneys") but, constrained by the AMA, did not take action to patent it.

Adrenalin was effective in the treatment of several ailments including asthma and, naturally, there was an attempt on its patent. In 1903, Parke-Davis sued H. K. Mulford Company for infringement when it produced and sold Adrin. But Mulford stood its ground arguing that their product was different and that, in any event, nature cannot be patented. In 1911, eight years later, Judge Learned Hand finally upheld the patent in part because there were no rules prohibiting the patenting of purified natural substances. As well, in the written ruling, the judge acknowledged that intravenous use of "the old dried glands" was a dangerous choice and that Takamine's invention was safer and it deserved support:

> Even if it were merely an extracted product without change, there is no rule that such products are not patentable. Takamine [the inventor] was the first to make it available for any use by removing it from the other gland-tissue in which it was found, and, while it is of course possible logically to call this a purification of the principle, it became for every practical purpose a new thing commercially and therapeutically. That was a good ground for a patent.[25]

Adrenaline or epinephrine increases heart rate and constricts blood vessels, thereby raising blood pressure. In 1903, researchers reported that injected adrenaline in the treatment of asthma reduced inflammation and provided instant if temporary relief.[26] With this success, researchers went on to vaporize adrenaline with oxygen, creating a convenient aerosol.[27]

The chemical operations of allergy took another lucrative leap forward in the discovery of histamine, histamine receptors, and antihistamines.

Pharmacologist Henry Dale (1875–1968) isolated histamine from mold and explored the essential actions of the chemical in the gut, respiratory tract, the heart, and in allergies. In 1927, Dale and his colleagues isolated the histamine from animal tissue samples and in 1937, found that adrenolytic benzodioxan could block the chemical in guinea pigs.[28]

Building on these discoveries, American chemist George Rieveschl (1916–2007) created a compound called diphenhydramine that had fewer side effects including reduced drowsiness. Diphenhydramine was renamed Benadryl™ after Rieveschl patented and licensed the product to Parke-Davis in 1946. Rieveschl received 5 percent royalty on Benadryl sales earning him $6 million a year by the early 1960s.[29]

CHE GUEVARA'S PUFFER

Argentine-born revolutionary Che Guevara (1928–1967) suffered from acute attacks of asthma throughout his life. "His chest sunken, deformed" from coughing and violent spasms that were often exercise induced; Che relied heavily on inhalers and epinephrine injections to recover.[30] A *TIME* magazine cover story from 1960 suggested a cause for the asthma—to toughen up his premature and sickly son, Che's father would expose him to the cold:

> Che was plunged into bathtubs of cold water and doused under icy showers. He developed a persistent cough and later serious allergic asthma.[31]

Che's condition inspired a natural interest in medicine, which he studied with the intention of becoming an allergist—he became a MD in 1953.[32] But as a revolutionary in 1957, Che continued to experience allergic reactions to mosquito venom that left large "cysts" as well as regular asthma attacks:

> The asthma was so strong it didn't let me advance. . . . I made it, but it, but with such an asthma attack that every single step was difficult . . . I had to make a decision because it was impossible for me to go on without at least buying medicines.[33]

Portable inhaler canisters with valves and measured doses of new anti-inflammatory steroids and bronchodilators were developed in the 1950s.[34] By 1961, Che's puffer likely contained a form of cortisone—a new treatment with side effects such as the telltale round face and weight gain, both of which were noted by his biographers.[35]

These convenient inhalers with new asthma drugs were prescribed liberally in the western world. Coincidental with the increased use of inhalers containing isoproterenol, however, there was a mysterious epidemic of asthma deaths in England and Wales starting in 1960 that peaked around 1968 (a year after Che's summary execution in Bolivia). The same or worse increase in asthma deaths in this period was observed in Ireland, Australia, New Zealand, and Norway.

It took four more years for the mystery to be solved: the approved concentration of the inhaled asthma drug was five times higher in the devices used in the affected countries—this compared with the United States or Canada and presumably also South America. The iatrogenic nature of the epidemic was discovered by Dr. Paul Stolley of Johns Hopkins. He published his conclusions in 1972:

> At least 3,500 asthmatics—most of them below the age of thirty-five—died suddenly during the 1960s in Britain alone. In children between the ages of ten and fourteen, asthma had become the fourth leading cause of death. It was the worst therapeutic drug disaster on record. There's nothing else—not even thalidomide—that ranks with it.[36]

PUTTING PANDORA BACK IN THE BOX: ANTI-ANAPHYLAXIS

As a child, allergist Robert Cooke (1880–1959) experienced asthma attacks to farm animals. By 1915, fourteen years after Richet "discovered" anaphylaxis through vaccination experiments, Cooke and colleagues tried to reverse the condition through the same means in "anti-anaphylaxis" or "desensitization" experiments:

> While the recognition of protein sensitization in the human is undoubtedly an advance, we still have no conception of the reason why or how a certain group of individuals become and remain sensitized while the deliberate inoculation of foreign protein in other persons leaves them eventually, to all intents and purposes, as unresponsive as thought they were never sensitized."[37]

Cooke injected 140 people with small and increasing linear doses of a pollen solution over two months before hay-fever season. During the season, shots continued every week to two weeks for a total of ten or twelve. Although Cooke did not call this a cure because symptoms returned the next year, it provided sufficient relief for some so desensitization injections were soon manufactured and sold.

Mark Jackson explains in *Allergy* that British physician Leonard Noon (1877–1913) began a method of planting, picking, drying, and extracting pollens in a standardized manner—a method continued by a pollenarium in England from which injectable preparations were made.

Supported financially by Parke-Davis, production of these desensitization injections made their way to market in the form of Pollaccine. A 1925 article reported on the success of Pollaccine when using the "ophthalmic method," injecting the desensitization vaccine into the eye.[38] In this case, the wrong dose resulted in a severe hay-fever attack in the allergic subject. However, adjusting the doses resulted in abatement of symptoms.

Allergy relief, however, was not always possible with this treatment. Finding the threshold of tolerance through immunotherapy was a problem for those who are "highly sensitized," allergist Warren Vaughan warned in his *Primer of Allergy.*[39] Indeed, while allergy shots became standard practice for allergists and many seasonal sufferers, they were not appropriate for peanut allergies. Clinical research with injected immunotherapy for life-threatening peanut allergy were shut down after significant reactions and at least one death in 1991 (see chapter 1).

An understanding of allergies and anaphylaxis, including testing and treatments, unfolded slowly through the twentieth century:

- 1918: Eczema was linked to food and environmental allergies[40]
- 1923: Cooke and Arthur Cola (1875-1959) coined the term atopy meaning "strange disease" to describe a person with multiple allergies, asthma, and eczema
- 1924: Skin prick test SPT technique used, became standard practice in 1960s
- 1935: Links were made between foods and pollen allergies (oral allergy syndrome) one triggering the other[41 42]
- 1953: Mast cells were identified
- 1963: Allergy classified by four types: anaphylactic, autoimmune, immune complex, and delayed

- 1966: The antibody immunoglobulin epsilon IgE was identified
- 1970: Leukotrienes were identified
- 1973: First formal study of peanut allergic children
- 1974: RAST technology for measuring IgE antibody levels in a blood sample
- 1980: Epipen introduced

ALLERGY'S BATTLEFIELD

Anyone who has experienced an anaphylactic reaction (or seen one) knows the debt of gratitude owed to emergency care workers. Benadryl, nebulizers, and epinephrine can arrest a reaction but as the drugs are metabolized, there can be a biphasic response with a return of symptoms. The drugs are readministered until the reaction is under control. Western medicine is at its best in a crisis.

Arguably, emergency medicine grew from the battlefield with rapid transport, triage, and emergency interventions. Through the early twentieth century, rotating on-call physicians at hospitals managed emergencies in coordination with ambulance services provided by funeral home directors and hearses. Specialized training in emergency medicine was established through the 1960s and 1970s—at this time, in comparison, battlefield medicine in the Vietnam War highlighted the weakness of civilian care, which was soon to improve.[43]

Through the twentieth century, ER care for reactions to drugs, vaccines, and sera were far more common than reactions to foods.

Serum sickness, starting in 1891 from the first anti-toxin sera for diphtheria, caused systemic reactions for many years—although primary research has not been conducted to know how many died. Reactions to aspirin began shortly after the drug was introduced in 1897[44] and, between 1912 and 1928, reactions to phenobarbital occurred in about 3% of those exposed to it. Sulfonamides were "highly sensitizing" in the late 1930s, and after WWII a tide of people became reactive to penicillin reminiscent of the days of epidemic serum sickness (see chapter 5).

In the last decades of the twentieth century, allergy had become an expensive health concern. In the United States, by the 1980s allergies had a price tag of $1.5 billion per year in medication, hospitalization, and services.[45] By 2013, that number had ballooned to $4.3 billion.[46] This included three hundred thousand ER visits for children and 3.6 million prescriptions for EpiPens.[47]

Patented in 1977 and brought to market in 1980, the EpiPen was designed originally for the US military as a lifesaving battlefield device. The civilian application of this portable, spring-loaded autoinjector of epinephrine has made it ubiquitous and lucrative. In 2011, following a tragic death of a child at school for whom an autoinjector was not available, Federal Bill S. 1884 provided "incentives to require elementary and secondary schools to maintain and permit school personnel to administer, epinephrine at schools."

There are 98,817 US public schools—the possible over-stocking of schools with autoinjectors is good news for parents with allergic children who are concerned that EMS may not arrive in time or if they are simply unable to afford the devices.

The soaring price of the EpiPen became a US national scandal in 2016 when Mylan, licensed to make and market the device, increased prices to about $600 for a two-pack—which is replaced annually. Possible gross revenue at these prices for the 3.6 million prescriptions alone sent Mylan shares north until August 2016 when the company's CEO was asked to defend the price hike before a House committee. There are no regulations on drug pricing in the United States, and without much competition Mylan was able to squeeze a fearful market reliant on the device.

While those with severe allergies—and their parents—are grateful for these lifesaving drugs; they are effectively tied to them forever. The notion of a cure is not the goal of the drug companies, but rather ongoing and costly management of allergy for the lifespan of the consumer.

THE ALLERGY FIX

By 2001, the primary cause of the allergy epidemic in infants and children was well known—it was and is an externalized cost of vaccination.[48] Allergists afraid of reprisals, loss of reputations, and jobs have suppressed warnings to parents. This has quickly deepened the crisis of severe allergies in children.

By 2009, the economy of the allergy epidemic and autoimmune illnesses in children have become so lucrative, as mentioned in the introduction, that one market analyst suggested that an autoimmune index would be a great tool for pharmaceutical investors. In "Save the Children (and Make Money)" published in the *Wall Street Journal*, the analyst seemed unaware of the irony of his own observation that pharmaceuticals were both the cause and "cure" of the epidemic:

> The increase in autoimmune illnesses and allergies in children may be due to high
> exposure to antibiotics and vaccines at an early age, preventing infections but also

inhibiting the body's ability to develop immunity to later infections.[49]

The lucrative relationship of scientist and pharmaceutical corporation in patented allergy medicines that began in the early twentieth century became a frenzied race to conquer symptoms, to destroy IgE, reprogram cells, and perform immunotherapy on atopic infants. These late-twentieth- and twenty-first–century treatments are framed by desperation, fear, and confusion on the part of parents and greed masked as concern on the part of allergists who persist in their bemused silence about the iatrogenic roots of the epidemic.

The war on IgE—attempts to block it, bind it, tag it with a virus, and kill it—began in 1996 with injected TNX-901 followed by Xolair (omalizumab) an anti-IgE antibody (humanized IgG) that inhibits the binding of IgE to receptors on mast cells and basophils. Adverse effects include anaphylaxis. The monthly cost of the drug is about $1,000. In 2009, 10% of children had asthma, for which Xolair was approved, according the American Academy of Allergy Asthma and Immunology.

An IgE epitope antigen using a hepatitis B virus protein as a carrier was designed to induce antibodies against a portion of the IgE molecule. This vaccine targets and destroys the IgE.[50] Other vaccines with a similar action use killed or inactivated vaccinia virus (smallpox) or tetanus toxoid to target and destroy IgE expressed by B cells. This vaccine can be used prophylactically or therapeutically.[51] A patent for this "anti-allergy" vaccine was granted in 2016.

In the war on IgE, researchers assumed that this annoying antibody was not needed for anything else. And yet, Margie Profet in *The Function of Allergy* (1991) offered that allergy as an evolved means of quickly removing a perceived toxin from the body, has a role to play in preventing cancer. A 2013 article highlighted that possibility suggesting that "IgE could have evolved because it functions also as a tumor surveillant."[52]

In the twenty-first century, immunotherapy pioneered for environmental allergies in the twentieth century was redeveloped for food allergies using controlled dose skin patches, capsules, and liquids.

DBV Technologies' peel-and-stick skin-arm patch for peanut allergy employs an "electrospray" that "sprays a liquid solution of electrically charged proteins onto the patch's backing." This solution contains the peanut allergen that is delivered through intact skin. The DBV web site calls this technology "highly scalable." A 2016 clinical study of seventy-four peanut allergic patients over fifty-two weeks, using two different doses, indicated a 48% and 45.8% success rate in a ten-fold increase in tolerance to peanut. The placebo group saw a 12% success rate. Side effects of the patch included hives and blisters.[53]

Oral immunotherapy (OIT) for peanut was originally dose controlled by allergists in their offices—ground peanut flour was measured and with tiny, but increasing doses created tolerance to the food in some children. The patient, however, must continue to consume the food forever on a regular basis to maintain this tolerance. But the treatment may work better, claimed a consumer magazine and doctors, if the treatment is given to infants, "the younger the better."[54]

OIT received a boost in popularity following the five-year LEAP study published in 2015. The LEAP study (Learn Early About Peanut Allergy) was created in 2010 to find "how to best prevent peanut allergy" in infants. But this was not a study about causes. The study's purpose was to prove the efficacy of infant oral immunotherapy in suppressing sensitization to peanut.

As described in chapter 2, children in the study deemed at high risk because they already had a severe egg allergy or eczema were as young as four months of age. One group was fed regular doses of peanut, another exposed randomly to the food. As anticipated, sensitization to peanut was suppressed in many children in the dosed OIT group. This proved again that controlled immunotherapy can promote tolerance (permanence was not established, however). They also showed that a major risk factor for developing peanut allergy is allergy and atopy.

But what was causing the severe allergies in the infants that made them at risk for peanut allergy? This linchpin question was left dangling and unanswered following the LEAP research. What remained was an opportunity for packaged oral immunotherapy liquids and capsules now poised to become a "normal" prophylactic for infants.

And yet, highly sensitive children cannot participate in OIT—the treatment has also been known to trigger EoE, esophageal eosinophilia, and chronic strangling inflammation of the esophagus that limits the ability to swallow.[55]

In 2016 came news of a therapy that manipulates another player in the allergic reaction—dendritic cells. These immune cells at the top of the allergic pathway send signals that can turn off reactive cells further downstream. The treatment involves producing dendritic cells that have been exposed to a mixture retinoic acid and allergens like peanut. The "mature retinoic acid-skewed dendritic cells" were injected into peanut allergic mice and found to reduce reactivity to oral challenge by 84% to 90%. Forkhead box P3 (Foxp3) regulatory T cells are believed to play a role in down-regulating the allergic response.[56] The treatment in mice resulted also in reduced allergen specific IgE and IgG levels.

Unique among the western allergy treatments is an "outsider," traditional Chinese medicine (TCM) herbal therapy. Dr. Xiu-Min Li, now in New York City but trained in China, found that a two-thousand-year-old remedy for parasites, Wu-Mei-Wan, blocked the peanut allergy in mice after seven weeks of treatment. Even five weeks after therapy there was no sign of a reaction.[57] Transferring a treatment from East to the West, however, meant it had to be scalable—it had to be mass produced in a one-size-fits all product. Food Allergy Herbal Formulae, FAHF1 and FAHF2 herbal combinations, were patented but in human clinical trials met an obstacle—not because of possible efficacy but because of compliance issues: six tablets of pressed herbs were consumed three times daily for six months. Swallowing that much herbal product proved to be a challenge.

Dr. Li has had success in her private clinic with tailored treatments involving herbal skin creams, drinks, pills, and bath powders that detoxify and calm the body over a period of two to three years. Her successes and challenges have been reported anecdotally through social media.

THE GHOST IN THE ALLERGY MACHINE

> But what emerged at the beginning of the twentieth century, was the fact that medicine could be dangerous, not through its ignorance and falseness, but through its knowledge, precisely because it was a science.
>
> Michel Foucault, "The Crisis of Medicine or
> the Crisis of Anti-Medicine?" 1976 [58]

The Cartesian mechanist view of the body has ruled the western approach to human health—for better and worse. In fact, Cartesian dualism that separates mind from the physical body is a "big mistake," stated philosopher Gilbert Ryle in *The Concept of Mind*.[59] With "deliberate abusiveness," Ryle (1900–1976) mocks the Cartesian doctrine, calling it "the dogma of the ghost in the machine." It is ridiculous that the means of interaction between the mind and physical reality within the doctrine is left as an unknowable, as a ghost in the mechanical body.

In the management of the body with allergy, specifically, the clock-body view has led to some important discoveries—adrenaline, histamine, and antihistamines. But nothing in western medicine has ever cured allergy and likely never will because it is rooted in a flawed doctrine. To quote Foucault, from *Birth of the Clinic*:

> That which is not on the scale of the gaze falls outside the domain of possible knowledge.

Even TCM, which is a more holistic approach using the synergistic effect of herbal combinations that has been known for thousands of years, still leaves the mind, its levels, its belief, and its consciousness out of the treatment.

Consciousness cannot be categorized, quantified, or dissected. For example, we know that histamine once released causes leaking of blood vessels and inflammation—but we don't know why. How does histamine "know" how to do what it does? How does the liver, with more than three hundred functions, know how to perform methylation as distinct from sulfation with such precision each and every time for years on end? And when something goes wrong, we might ask what aspect of consciousness is communicating and reflecting filtered perceptions of outer experiences on our inner workings?

Epigenetics is the study of environmental influences on genetic expression. Change the environment and you change the cell, explains biologist Bruce Lipton (b. 1944). Each of our fifty trillion cells is an individual with the potential to become anything. What determines its fate is the environment. In *The Wisdom of Your Cells* (2007), Lipton explains that it is perception of the environment that communicates to the cell membrane where there are "over a hundred thousand different switches prepared to respond to a massive variety of environmental signals." Nocebo and placebo responses to the environment are examples of this phenomenon, where what you believe manifests physically (see chapter 2). And so, to recover from allergy, we may need to learn how to step out of our programmed thoughts and fears and question what we have been taught and believe about manifestations of allergy and disease.

And what would Richet have to say about this idea—the man who after discovering anaphylaxis went on to discover ectoplasm? Not entirely tethered to the medical model, Richet sought for thirty years to prove the existence of a sixth sense, a paranormal communication he had glimpsed between people, living and dead. And yet, in the "real" world, Richet supported the medicalization of society despite the adverse vaccination outcome of anaphylaxis. He explained in his Nobel acceptance speech in 1913:

> Anaphylaxis is thus necessary to the species, often to the detriment of the individual. The individual may perish, but this does not matter. The species must at all times retain its organic integrity. Anaphylaxis defends the species against the peril of adulteration.

In other words, anaphylaxis weeds out the weak—which is a view little different from that of the doctor today who also knows vaccination creates anaphylaxis and remains silent, believing that it is a cost unwary members of the herd must pay.

But this medical violence against children cannot continue forever. When enough children have been made allergic and the parent and grown child understand the game in which they have been made pawns, there will be a revolution. The revolution may be quiet as is occurring in Canada—deeply concerned parents are turning away from vaccination. In response, legislative changes in Alberta and Ontario will force parents into classrooms to consume unbalanced government lectures on the good of vaccination. The Canadian Medical Association in 2016 passed a resolution supporting mandatory vaccination. In the United States in 2016, the very vocal revolution against mandatory vaccination is moving into another dimension after the election of a new president who has spoken openly about vaccine injury.

The authority of medicine rests on so-called objective scientific truth. Medicine assumes its discoveries to be fact rather than a reformulation of knowledge, classification, and reclassification of the body, its symptoms, and its treatment—which in *materia medica* is centuries old. We look back on the tortuous treatment of arsenic cream, bleeding, purges, inhalants, injections, and in this distance of one hundred years, can see how nothing has changed. Yes, there have been valuable discoveries but the risk benefit balance has upended. The most vulnerable members of society are experiencing an iatrogenic epidemic of unprecedented proportions.

But now, it comes down to the parents, to the mother. The child is protected and represented by the mother who may be persuaded to remain silent by the carrot of "cure," the allergy off-switch—the part that can be taken out or "fixed" so the body can return to normal. In other words, the mother may be silent about causes for fear of angering her only hope of recovering her child. How many allergy mothers are there who know what is happening and are willing to speak out?

Here is an opportunity to recognize where being female may intersect unfavorably with medicine, while at the same time knowing there is nothing more powerful than turning away and saying no.

APPENDIX

The following figures reveal an upward trend of peanut allergy in children living in affected countries.

AFRICA

- In 2013, reactions to peanut in 1.5% and sensitization in 17.5% of Ghanaian schoolchildren.[1] In 2006, Gideon Lack noted in a speech mentioned in the British Medical Journal the 0% incidence of peanut allergy in Sub-Saharan Africa suggesting the reason being the early consumption of peanuts at weaning and beyond. Either he was mistaken or the phenomenon of peanut allergy grew rapidly.[2] There was serologic evidence of sensitivity in 5% of Xhosan children in Cape Town (2007),[3] but with no reported cases of anaphylaxis. By 2011 another study of Xhosan children in an urban high school showed 1.9% sensitized and reacting to peanut.[4]

AUSTRALIAN CAPITAL TERRITORY (ACT), AUSTRALIA

- Of school-entrant ACT children, 2% (2009) were confirmed by diagnostic test to be peanut allergic.[5] ACT is a self-governing state with the highest density population and smallest area at 910 square miles. Within it is the national capital, Canberra. According to the Australasian Society of Clinical Immunology and Allergy, 1.15% of ACT children born in 2004 were peanut allergic, compared to 0.47% of those born in 1995.[6] National figures are 0.71% (2001)[7] and 0.5% (1995).[8] Children make up 26% of the Australian population. Therefore, in 2009 of almost 22 million Australians, there were about 5.7 million children, 114,400 of whom were peanut allergic.

MELBOURNE, AUSTRALIA

- 3% of children were found to be allergic just to peanut in Melbourne in a 2011 published study.[9]

TASMANIA, AUSTRALIA

- This Australian island and state's figures are 1.11% in 2009[10] and 0% in 2001.[11] Of a population-based cohort of 456 Tasmanian children aged seven to eight years, none reacted to a peanut skin prick test in 2001. By 2009, 1.11% were reactive to peanut.

MONTREAL, CANADA

- 1.21% to 2.33% of children in a Canadian nation-wide survey in 2009 were found to be peanut allergic.[12] Of children under nine in Montreal, Canada, 1.71% or more (2007) were peanut allergic.[13] In 2009 there were 7.8534 million children in Canada under nineteen. Therefore, as many as 183,000 children were peanut allergic.

NORTHEASTERN EUROPE

- Geographically close countries in northeastern Europe—Estonia, Lithuania, and Russia—appear to have a very low prevalence of peanut allergy[14]
- Data are limited for this area. A study of a Lithuanian birth cohort born between 2006 and 2007 found 2.8% of 12 month olds were sensitized to foods primarily egg and dairy. Peanut allergy was low being found in two from a group of 1553 children.[15]
- A 2014 published study of peanut allergy in children from the Tomsk Region of Russia indicated that just .08% of children were reactive to the food.[16]
- It is worth noting that the health infrastructure of Russia appears to have been weak with allergy and 'weakness' being a contraindication to immunization until about 1996. De-worming is an ongoing initiative. The Hib B vaccine was introduced by the Russian Ministry of Health only after 2010. http://rostropovich.org.

FRANCE

- Of children under fifteen in France, 0.45% or more (2000) were peanut allergic.[17]

GERMANY

- No firm statistics are available, although peanut allergy seems of limited significance. In a 2005 analysis of physician-reported cases of 103 anaphylactic children in Germany, foods were the most frequent cause of the reaction (57%, and of this number 20% to peanut) followed by insect stings (13%) and immunotherapy injections (12%). Peanuts and tree nuts were the foods most frequently causing the reactions.[18] In a 2004 study of food allergy in Berlin children and teens, there appeared to be no self-reported symptoms brought on by peanut.[19]

HONG KONG

- Of Chinese children aged two to seven living in Hong Kong, 0.57% to 1%[20] were reactive to peanut (2009). A EuroPrevall Prague report indicated that 0.7% of Hong Kong's study participants were peanut allergic (2008). Studies published in 1994[21] and 1999[22] concluded that sensitization to peanut was rare in Chinese children living in Hong Kong. In fact, it seemed rare to find peanut allergy at all in Southeast Asia.[23] Subsequent reports in 2001/2002 reiterated that while the per capita consumption of peanuts in China is similar to that in the United States, peanut allergy was rare in China. By 2008, 0.57 to 1% of Chinese children were reacting to peanut. Chinese American children living in the United States had an incidence of peanut allergy similar to that of the general US population (2001).[24]

INDIA

- Limited data are available on peanut allergy in India although food allergy in general is believed to be increasing. There are no recent studies of peanut allergy.[25]

ISRAEL

- .6% (2012) Jewish Israeli children aged 13-14 allergic to peanut.[26] This is up from .17% (2002).[27]
- In the same country, 2.5% (2012) of Arab Israeli 13-14 year old children were peanut allergic.

JAPAN

- In 2003, population-based prevalence figures for food allergy in Japan were apparently unavailable.[28] The most common food allergen among Japanese children was hen's egg, followed by cow's milk and then wheat. These three food allergens accounted for 60% of pediatric food allergy. Peanut allergy appears generally not to be a concern.

NORWAY AND DENMARK

- In 2005, 0.5% of Danish adolescents reacted to peanuts.[29] In 2001, the numbers of peanut-allergic children in Norway and Denmark were believed to be very low.[30]

SINGAPORE

- Of children aged five to twelve living in Singapore, 1.08%–1.35% were reactive to peanut in 2007.[31] A 1997 study had alluded to reports of peanut allergy from several Asian centers including Singapore, the Philippines, Malaysia, Indonesia, Japan, Beijing, Hong Kong, and Taiwan.[32] Sensitization to peanut was second to shellfish in cohort under five according to a National University of Singapore professor (2005). Significantly, although children were sensitized to peanut, there were no reported cases of anaphylaxis. The reason for this was not known although lack of exposure to peanuts was not a factor.[33] However, by 2007, a three-year study revealed a "worrying trend" of peanut reactivity in Asian children living in Singapore (Chinese, Malay, Indian, and Eurasian ethnic groups).[34] Peanut allergy was found in 27.3% of food-allergic children.

SWEDEN

- Of children under six in Sweden, 1.2% or more (1998) were reactive to peanut.[35] In 2000, 2.139 million people were under age nineteen. Therefore, 25,668 children were allergic to peanuts in 1998.

UNITED KINGDOM

- A total 1.8% of schoolchildren were allergic to peanuts in 2007.[36] In 2008, there were 11.5 million children under sixteen. Therefore, an estimated 207,000 children in the United Kingdom were allergic to peanuts. Statistics have ranged from 3% to 1% in a study of 70 children (1.43%).[37]

UNITED STATES

- 2% - 2.8% or 1.5 to 2 million peanut allergic children in 2010 was an apparent increase from a 2008 study in which 1.4% children were found to be allergic.[38] 0.8% children under eighteen were reactive to peanut in 2002.[40]

NOTES

THE PROBLEM OF PEANUT ALLERGY

1. See appendix.
2. "Rate of childhood peanut allergies more than tripled from 1997 to 2008," *ScienceDaily* (May 13, 2010), www.sciencedaily.com/releases/2010/05/10051211 2320.htm.
3. The World Health Organization's Codex Alimentarius Commission (est. 1963) created a list of critical food allergens in 1996: peanut, tree nut, fish, shellfish, wheat, soy, dairy, egg. These eight account for about 90% of all food reactions.
4. The peanut epitopes are Ara h 1, Ara h2 (5 subtypes), Ara h3 through 8, Ara h Agglutinin, Ara h LTP, Ara h Oleosin, and Ara h T1.
5. R. Fischer et al., "Oral and nasal sensitization promote distinct Immune responses and lung reactivity in mouse model of peanut allergy," *American Journal of Pathology* 16, no. 6 (Dec. 2005): 1,621–1,630; and C. A. Coop et al., "Anaphylaxis from the influenza virus vaccine," *International Archives of Allergy and Immunology* 146, no. 1 (2008): 85–8.
6. Margie Profet, "The Function of Allergy: Immunological Defense against Toxins," *The Quarterly Review of Biology* 66, no. 1 (March 1991): 23–62.
7. H. Zinsser, T. Tamiya, "An experimental analysis of bacterial allergy," *The Journal of Experimental Medicine* 44 (1926): 753–776; and V. I. Klots, "The case of allergy to cholera vaccine," *Foreign Technology Division Wright Patterson AFB, Ohio, Defense Technical Information Center* (Oct. 9, 1974), http://oai.dtic.mil/oai/oai?ver b=getRecord&metadataPrefix=html&identifier=ADA000172.
8. M. Modrzynski et al., "The occurrence of food allergy and bacterial allergy in children with tonsilar hypertrophy," *Przegl Lek* 61,no. 12 (2004):1330–3.
9. C. J. Hackett, D. A. Ham (ed.), *Vaccine adjuvants: immunological and clinical principals* (Humana Press, 2006): 139.
10. Profet, "The Function of Allergy," 23–62.

11. H. Kuno-Sakai, M. Kimura, "Removal of gelatin from live vaccines and DTaP— an ultimate solution for vaccine-related gelatin allergy," *Biologicals* 31 (2003): 245–249.

12. I. N. Glaspole et al., "Anaphylaxis to lemon soap: citrus seed and peanut allergen cross-reactivity," *Annals of Allergy, Asthma and Immunology* 98, no. 3 (March 2007): 286–9.

13. Quoted in Alice Park, "The Truth About Vaccines," *Time* (Canadian Edition, June 2, 2008): 34.

14. M. R. Odent, "Long term effects of early vaccinations," *Primal Health Research Newsletter* 2, no. 1 (1994): 6.

15. G. W. Ewing, "What is regressive autism and why does it occur? Is it the consequence of multi-system dysfunction affecting the elimination of heavy metals and the ability to regulate neural temperature?" *North American Journal of Medical Sciences* 1, no. 2 (July 2009): 34. See also A. W. Taylor-Robinson, "Multiple vaccination effects on atopy," *Allergy* 54 (April 1999): 398–399; and H. Albonico et al., "The immunization campaign against measles, mumps and rubella—coercion leading to a realm of uncertainty: medical objections to a continued MMR immunization campaign in Switzerland," *The Journal of the American Medical Association* 9, 1 (1992).

16. James Altucher, "Save the children (and make money)," *The Wall Street Journal* (August 10, 2009). http://online.wsj.com/article/SB12499239038 7319939.html.

CHAPTER 1: FROM IDIOSYNCRASY TO MULTIBILLION-DOLLAR INDUSTRY

1. "Doctor nearly dies of salted peanuts," *The New York Times*, Books Section, (Mon., Dec. 20, 1954) 31.

2. George W. Gray, "Allergy, protection gone wild," *Harper's Magazine* rerun in the *Milwaukee Journal* (Sat., Jan. 1, 1939).

3. "Doctor finds a new drug to treat allergies," *Chicago Tribune* (April 17, 1949).

4. *Allergy to Cottonseed and Other Oilseeds and Their Edible Derivatives. Excerpts from Testimony before the Administrator, Federal Security Agency, in the matter of fixing and establishing definitions and standards of identity for mayonnaise, French dressing, and related salad dressings* (U.S. Federal Security Agency and the National Cottonseed Products Association, 1948). This book documents public hearings held in Washington (Nov. 1947–Jan. 1948) in which doctors and cottonseed oil workers testified on the safety of refined cottonseed oil and lack of standards in the crushing industry, which led to cross contamination of many oils subsequently used in various processed foods. Articles on "hypersensitivity" and allergy to

cottonseed appeared in the 1940s and '50s in *Pediatrics, Annals of Allergy, Journal of American Medical Association, Acta allergologica.*

5.   Cottonseed allergy and anaphylaxis were reported in Judy E. Perkin (ed.), *Food allergies and adverse reactions* (Aspen, 1990) 57. Cottonseed oil is used in medications and foods including mayonnaise, fried potato chips, and oil-packed tuna. Cottonseed flour may be found in baked goods, candy, spices, cream substitutes, and processed meats.

6.   G. Hildick-Smith et al., "Penicillin Regimens in Pediatric Practice: Study of Blood Levels," *Pediatrics* (Jan. 1950): 97–113. This article reports that the Romansky formula created sensitivity to peanut oil in a study of children at the Children's Hospital of Philadelphia. See also P. C. Trussell et al., "Duration of Effective Blood levels following administration of penicillin in peanut oil and beeswax," *Canadian Medical Association Journal* 57 (Oct. 1947): 387; and R. V. Platou et al., "Round Table Discussion on Antibiotics," *Pediatrics* (Feb. 1948).

7.   A. P. Black, "A new diagnostic method in allergic disease," *Pediatrics* 17 (May 1956): 716–724; S. Goldman et al., "Milk Allergy," *Pediatrics* 32 (Sept. 1963): 425–443; and W. G. Crook et al., "Systemic Manifestations Due to Allergy: Report on Fifty Patients," *Pediatrics* 27 (May 1961): 790–799. Both articles observe an increase in peanut and food allergy in children.

8.   Jean Mayer, "Better labeling laws are needed," *Pittsburgh Post-Gazette* (June 5, 1972) 12.

9.   S. A. Bock, F. M. Atkins, "The natural history of peanut allergy," *The Journal of Allergy and Clinical Immunology* 83, no. 5 (June 1, 1989): 900–4. Bock and others pioneered the use of the double-blind placebo-controlled food challenge (DBPCFC).

10.   F. Speer, "Multiple food allergy," *Annals of Allergy* 34, no. 2 (Feb. 1975): 71–6. Further studies indicated that peanut allergic children typically had multiple food allergies.

11.   www.sarnoffendowment.org/about/history.cfm.

12.   "Candy kills peanut allergic youth," *The Spokesman-Review* (Spokane, Washington, Sept. 28, 1980).

13.   (UPI), "Allergy kills Brown student," *The New York Times* (June 5, 1986).

14.   "Stricken in the cabin," *Los Angeles Times* (April 1, 1988).

15.   Warren Vaughan, *Strange Malady, The Story of Allergy* (New York: Doubleday, Doran & Co., 1941): 111.

16.   "Bite of cake ends a boy's struggle for life," *Sacramento Bean* (Jan. 16, 1987); "Allergic reaction death," *Ocala* (Florida) *Star-Banner* (Jan. 16, 1987); "When food becomes poison," *The Ledger* (Sept. 10, 1987); and "A lot of food hazard hides in undercooked vittles," *The Courier* (Prescott, Arizona) (Oct. 28, 1986): "Every week brings reports of new dangers; a death from allergy."

17. "How to prevent severe allergic reactions," *St. Petersburg* (Florida) *Times* (July 21, 1988); "Those with deadly allergies need epinephrine," *The Ledger* (July 21, 1988); "Many treatments available for hives," *Chicago Tribune* (July 29, 1988); "Battling deadly allergies, stimulant epinephrine can help victims," *St. Petersburg* (Florida) *Times* (July 21, 1988); "Allergy-prone people advised on fast relief in simple kit," *Los Angeles Times* (July 24, 1988); "People with potentially deadly allergies require epinephrine," *Ludington* (Michigan) *Daily News* (Sept. 9, 1988).

18. "When your immune system panics, anaphylaxis, severe allergic reaction," *The Saturday Evening Post* (Oct. 1, 1989); "Listing ingredients for allergy sufferers," *St. Louis Post-Dispatch* (Jan. 9, 1989) reflects on 1986 peanut-chili death; "Children at risk from things safe for adults," *Los Angeles Daily News* (April 3, 1989); "Body and mind: Backward protection," *The New York Times* (July 2, 1989); "Allergy guide makes shopping for special foods easier," *The Gazette* (Colorado Springs, Feb. 15, 1989).

19. "Food allergies: Cause for concern or over-diagnosed malady?" *Environmental Nutrition* (Nov. 1, 1989).

20. S. A. Bock et al., "Fatalities due to anaphylactic reactions to food," *Journal of Allergy and Clinical Immun.* 107, no. 1 (Jan. 2001): 191–93; A. M. Barnam, S. L. Lukacs, "Food allergy among US children: Trends in prevalence and hospitalizations," *National Centre for Health Statistics*, CDC (Oct. 22, 2008). This trend continued. Four in every 100 US children in 2008 had a severe food allergy.

21. R. J. Mullins, "Pediatric food allergy trends in a community-based specialist allergy practice, 1995–2006," *Medical Journal of Australia* 186, no. 12 (2007): 618–621.

22. Du Toit, et al., "Randomized trial of peanut consumption in infants at risk for peanut allergy," *The New England Journal of Medicine*, Vol. 372, No. 9 (Feb. 26, 2015): 803-813.

23. Y. Levy, et al., "Trends in adrenaline dispensing in Israel in 1997-2004," *Public Health*, Vol. 121, No. 2 (Feb., 2007): 14407. http://www.ncbi.nlm.nih.gov/pubmed/17161854.

24. V. Hoffer, et al., "Anaphylaxis in Israel, experience with 92 hospitalized children," *Pediatric Allergy and Immunology*, Vol. 22, No. 2 (March 2011):172-177. http://onlinelibrary.wiley.com/doi/10.1111/j.1399-3038.2010.00990.x/abstract.

25. Yael Graif, et al., "Association of food allergy and asthma severity and atopic diseases in Jewish and Arab adolescents," *Acta Paediatr,* 101 (10) (2012): 1083-8.

26. A. Sheik, "Life threatening allergy, an homage to Von Pirquet," *World Allergy Forum Symposium* (Sun. June 11, 2006). Lecture recorded in Vienna, Austria, www.worldallergy.org/educational_programs/world_allergy_forum/vienna2006/syllabus_book.pdf; and R. Gupta, A. Sheikh et al. "Increasing hospital admissions

for systemic allergic disorders in England: Analysis of national admissions data," *British Medical Journal* 327 (Nov. 2003): 1142–1143.

27. www.foodnavigator.com/Science-Nutrition/Peanut-allergies-rising-reveals-U.K.-study; and J. Grundy et al., "Rising prevalence of allergy to peanut in children: Data from 2 sequential cohorts," *Journal of Allergy and Clinical Immunology* 110, no. 5 (Nov. 2002).

28. "Parents warned of peanut risk to children," *The Independent* (United Kingdom, April 26, 1996); and "40,000 children in peril from peanuts; the growing taste that can kill," *Daily Mirror* (United Kingdom, April 2, 1996).

29. C. Thompson, "One bite and he dies," *Sunday Times* (London) *Magazine* (Oct. 19, 1997) 24–8; S. de Bruxelles, "Nuts led to death of allergic scientist," *The Times* (London, Nov. 21, 1997); D. Hide, "Fatal anaphylaxis due to food," *BMJ* 307 (27 Nov. 27, 1993): 1427; and E. S. K. Assem et al., "Anaphylaxis induced by peanuts," *BMJ* 307 (May 26, 1990): 1377.

30. www.foodnavigator.com/Science-Nutrition/Peanut-allergies-rising-reveals-U.K.-study; J. Grundy, Op. cit.

31. T. Burchill, "The rise of killer food," *The Times* (London), T2 (Jan. 22, 2002): 10.

32. L. Chiu et al. "Estimation of the sensitization rate to peanut by prick skin test in the general population: Results from the National Health and Nutrition Examination Survey, 1980–1994," *J Allergy Clin Immunol* 107 (2001): S192.

33. K. Beyer et al., "Effects of cooking methods on peanut allergenicity," *Journal of Allergy and Clinical Immunology* 107, no. 6 (June 2001): 1077–1081.

34. S. A. Bock et al., "Fatalities due to anaphylactic reactions to foods," *J. Allergy Clin. Immunol.* 107 (2001): 191–193.

35. "Experiment produces promising allergy therapy injections ease reaction to peanuts," *Charlotte Observer* (March 12, 1992).

36. A. Gosline, "Peanut allergy: Dining with death," *New Scientist* 25, no. 57, (June 21, 2006).

37. N. Moran, "Ultimate allergy shot. Innovation: British company boasts of a vaccine with huge potential," *The Independent* (London) (Jan. 29, 1995).

38. D. Hamilton, "Silent treatment, how Genentech, Novartis stifled a promising drug, biotech firm tried to pursue peanut-allergy injection, but contract got in way," *The Wall Street Journal* A1 (April 5, 2005).

39. E. Ostblom, et al., "Phenotypes of food hypersensitivity and development of allergic diseases during the first 8 years of life," *Clin Exp Allergy*, 38 (8) (2008): 1325-32.

40. Leon S. Kind, L. Roesner, "Enhanced susceptibility of pertussis inoculated mice to pollen extract," *Proc Soc Exp Biol Med.* 100, no. 4 (April 1959): 808–10.

41. C. Chang, R. Y. Gottshall, "Sensitization to ragweed pollen in Bordetella pertussis-infected or vaccine-injected mice," *Journal of Allergy and Clinical Immunology* 54, no. 1 (July 1974): 20–24.

42. R. Fischer et al., "Oral and Nasal Sensitization Promote distinct immune responses and reactivity in a mouse model of peanut allergy," *American Journal of Pathology* 167 (2005): 1621–1630.

43. "Center expands marketing of allergy product," *Health Industry Today* (July 1992).

44. In 1998, pharmaceutical giant Merck took a share in EpiPen sales through its ownership of Dey, L. P. EMI, an affiliate of Dey, L. P. became the exclusive distributor of EpiPen that was manufactured by Meridian Medical Technologies and marketed by King Pharmaceuticals a subsidiary of Meridian—Meridian was formed in 1996 by the merger of STI and Brunswick Biomedical. Dey assumed exclusive distribution rights in 2001. Majority of Dey Inc. was acquired in 1991 by Merck and then all of it by 1998. In 2008, 1.9 million EpiPens were sold in the United States, up more than 33% from 2003.

45. "Son's deadly allergy pits mom against school," *The Salt Lake Tribune* (April 4, 1994).

46. "Prestigious school rejects boy with peanut allergy," *Lexington* (Kentucky) *Herald-Leader* (April 15, 1995).

47. "Mom comes up with lifesaving badge," *The Orange County* (California) *Register* (May 5, 1994).

48. Wendy Harris, "Abnormal Response to Normal Things," *Professionally Speaking Magazine, Ontario College of Teachers* (Toronto, Sept. 2000).

49. "Goodbye to the Goober," *Newsweek* (Oct. 4, 1996).

50. Laura Lang, "Life threatening allergies spur peanut bans at Mass. Schools," *Education Week* (Nov. 6, 1996).

51. "Staple under fire: Kids allergies bring schools' ban on peanut butter," *Arizona Daily Star* (Sept. 23, 1996).

52. S. M. Fletcher, "Snack peanuts purchase pattern," *Journal of Agricultural and Applied Economics* (April 1, 2002).

53. Emmanuel Foko, *Transforming Mature Industries into growth industries: The case of U.S. peanuts* (Master of Agribusiness dissertation, Kansas State University, 2008).

54. "Group OKs GMO peanut research," *High Plains Journal* (Dec. 28, 2006). hpj.com.

55. Aaron Rowe, "Genetically modified peanuts could save lives," *Wired Science* (Nov. 30, 2008). www.wired.com/wiredscience/2008/11/peanuts-with-le/.

56. "NSW: Peanut allergy case ends in multimillion dollar settlement," *AAP General News* (Australia) (June 8, 2000).

57. The law is named for Sabrina Shannon, a twelve-year-old girl who died in 2003 from anaphylactic shock after consuming cafeteria french fries contaminated by cheese.

58. "Mr. Peanut goes to court," *Journal of Law and Health* (Cleveland Marshall College of Law, March 22, 1999).

59. "Bullies use peanut butter to threaten kids with allergies," *The Globe and Mail* (Canada, March 30, 2009).

60. "Man sentenced in peanut butter attack," *United Press International* (Dec. 27, 2008).

61. "Warning of nut allergy 'hysteria'," *BBC News* online (Dec. 10, 2008).

62. N. A. Christakis, "This allergy is just nuts," *British Medical Journal* (2008). This author is professor of Medical Sociology, Harvard Medical School.

63. "Call for specialist centres to tackle 'allergy epidemic'," *The Independent* (United Kingdom, Sept. 26, 2007).

64. "The Food Allergy & Anaphylaxis Network (FAAN) and Verus Pharmaceuticals work together to raise awareness of food allergies," *PR Newswire* (Oct. 4, 2007). Verus produces the portable epinephrine dispensing Twinject, a competitor to EpiPen.

65. C. A. Camargo et al., "Regional differences in EpiPen prescriptions in the United States," *The Journal of Allergy and Clinical Immunology* 120, no. 1 (July 2007): 131–136.

CHAPTER 2: RISK FACTORS

1. I. Dalal et al., "Food allergy is a matter of geography after all: Sesame as a major cause of severe IgE-mediated food allergic reactions among infants and young children in Israel," *European Journal of Allergy and Clinical Immunology* 57, no. 4 (March 2002): 362–365.

2. S. H. Sicherer et al. "Prevalence of peanut and tree nut allergy in the United States determined by means of a random digit dial telephone survey: A 5-year follow up study," *The Journal of Allergy and Clinical Immunology* 112, no. 6, (Dec. 2003): 1203–1207.

3. See appendix.

4. Y Hu, et al, "Comparison of food allergy prevalence among Chinese infants in Chongqing, 2009 versus 1999," *Pediatr Int*, 52 (2010): 820–824.

5. S. Maleki et al., "Is the low prevalence of peanut allergy in Israel due to hypoallergenic peanut products?" *J Allergy Clin Imunol* 115, 2 (Feb. 2005).

6. K. du Plessis, H. Steinman, "Practical aspects of adverse reactions to peanut," *Current Allergy & Clinical Immunology* 17, no. 1 (March 2004): 10–14.

7. Van Odijk, Op. cit.

8. Z. Kmietowicz, "Women warned to avoid peanuts during pregnancy and lactation," *BMJ* 316 (June 1998): 1926.

9. Ibid.

10. R. Hatahet, et al., "Sensibilisation aux allergens d'arachide chez les nourrissons de moins de quarter mois: À propos de 125 observations," *Revue Française d'ALlergologie et d'Immunologie Clinique* 34 (1994): 377–81.

11. P. W. Ewan, "Prevention of peanut allergy," *The Lancet* 352, no. 9129 (Aug. 1998): 741–2.

12. G. Lack et al., "Factors associated with the development of peanut allergy in childhood," *New England Journal of Medicine* 348 (2003): 977–85.

13. S. H. Sicherer et al., "Maternal consumption of peanut during pregnancy is associated with peanut sensitization in atopic infants," *The Journal of Allergy and Clinical Immunology* (June 2010) www.jacionline.org/article/S0091-6749(10)01334-5/ fulltext.

14. T. C. Liang, *Maternal Dietary Modification for Prevention of Food Sensitisation* (Master of Nutrition and Dietetics dissertation, University of Wollongong, 2007).

15. T. Dean, "Government advice on peanut avoidance during pregnancy: Is it followed correctly and what is the impact on sensitization?" *Journal of Human Nutrition and Dietetics* 20 (2007): 95–99.

16. A. Muraro et al. "Dietary prevention of allergic diseases in infants and small children part III," *Pediatric Allergy and Immunology* 15 (2004): 291–307.

17. D. Moneret-Vautrin et al., "Risk of milk formulas containing peanut oil contaminated with peanut allergens in infants with atopic dermatitis," *Pediatr Allergy Immunol* 5 (1994): 184–188; G. De Montis et al., "Sensitization to peanut and vitamin D oily preparations," *Lancet* 341 (1993): 1411; and A. Cantani, "Anaphylaxis from peanut oil in infant feedings and medications," *European Review of Medical and Pharmacological Sciences* 2 (1998): 203–206.

18. G. K. Appelt et al., "Breastfeeding and food avoidance are ineffective in preventing sensitization in high risk children," *The Journal of Allergy and Clinical Immunology* 113, no. 2 (2004): 299.

19. *Memorandum by European Academy of Allergology and Clinical Immunology, The United Kingdom Parliament, House of Lord, Science and Technology, Minutes Evidence* (2007).

20. G. Du Toit et al., "Early consumption of peanuts in infancy is associated with a low prevalence of peanut allergy," *Journal of Allergy and Clinical Immunology* 122 (Nov. 2008): 984–91.

21. I. Dalal et al. "The pattern of sesame sensitivity among infants and children," *Pediatr Allergy Immunol* 14, no. 4 (Aug. 2003): 312–6.

22. G. Du Toit, "Learning Early about peanut allergy, The LEAP study," *The Newsletter of the British Society for Allergy & Clinical Immunology* 8 (Autumn 2006): 6.

23. Du Toit, et al., "Randomized trial of peanut consumption in infants at risk for peanut allergy," *The New England Journal of Medicine*, Vol. 372, No. 9 (Feb. 26, 2015): 803–813.

24. Y. Levy, et al., "Trends in adrenaline dispensing in Israel in 1997-2004," *Public Health*, Vol. 121, No. 2 (Feb., 2007): 14407.

25. V. Hoffer, et al., "Anaphylaxis in Israel, experience with 92 hospitalized children," *Pediatric Allergy and Immunology*, Vol. 22, No. 2 (March 2011):172–177.

26. Yael Graif, et al., "Association of food allergy and asthma severity and atopic diseases in Jewish and Arab adolescents," *Acta Paediatr*, 101 (10) (2012): 1083–8.

27. www.leapstudy.co.uk/study_about.html

28. G. Du Toit, "Learning Early about Peanut Allergy, The LEAP Study," The Newsletter of the British Society for Allergy & Clinical Immunology 8 (Autumn 2006): 6.

29. J. Strid, et al., A novel model of sensitization and oral tolerance to peanut protein," *Immunology* 113, no. 3 (Nov. 2004): 293–303.

30. K. Bock, *Healing the New Childhood Epidemics, Autism, ADHD, Asthma and Allergies* (New York, Random House, 2007): 182.

31. H. A. Sampson, "Food allergy: When mucosal immunity goes wrong," *J Allergy Clin Immunol* 115, no. 1 (Jan. 2005): 139–141.

32. J. L. Hughes et al., "Peanut allergy and allergic airways inflammation," *Pediatr Allergy Immunol* 21, no. 8 (Dec. 2010): 1107–13.

33. "Allergy," *House of Lords, Science and Technology Committee, 6th Report of Session 2006-07*, I (Sept. 2007).

34. L. Miles, J. L. Buttriss, "Government advice revised, early life exposure to peanut no longer a risk factor for peanut allergy," *Nutrition Bulletin* 35, no. 3 (Sept. 2010): 240–244.

35. S. Sicherer et al., "Food hypersensitivity and atopic dermatitis: pathophysiology, epidemiology, diagnosis and management," *J Allergy Clin Immunol* 104, no. 3 (1999): S114–S122.

36. H. Sampson, "Managing peanut allergy," *BMJ* 312 (1996): 1050–1.

37. J. O'B Hourihane et al. "Peanut allergy in relation to heredity, maternal diet, and other atopic diseases: Results of a questionnaire survey, skin prick testing, and food challenges," *BMJ* 313 (Aug. 1996): 518–521.

38. D. J. Hill et al., "The frequency of food allergy in Australia and Asia," *Environmental Toxicology and Pharmacology* 4, no.1–2 (Nov. 1997): 101–110.

39. G. Du Toit, "Different prevalence of peanut allergy in children in Israel and U.K. is not due to differences in atopy," *Journal of Allergy and Clinical Immunology* 117, no. 2 (Feb. 2006): Supplement.

40. Prescott, S, Allen K., "Food Allergy: riding the second wave of the allergy epidemic, *Pediatric Allergy & Immunology*, 22 (2011):155-160.

41. T. Kemp T. et al., "Is infant immunization a risk factor for childhood asthma or allergy?" *Epidemiology* 8 (1997): 678–680.

42. M. Odent et al., "Pertussis vaccination and asthma: Is there a link?" *JAMA*, 272, 8 (Aug. 1994): 593. Quoted in A. Mercae, *From Immunology to social policy: Epistemology and ethics in the creation and administration of paediatric vaccines* (Dissertation, University of Tasmania, April 2003). http://eprints.utas.edu.au/31/1/ Arlette_Mercae_Thesis.pdf; M. Odent, E. Culpin, "Effect of immunization status on asthma prevalence," *The Lancet* 361, no. 9355 (Feb. 2003): 434; and H. Odelram et al., "Immunoglobulin E and G responses to pertussis toxin after booster immunization in relation to atopy, local reactions and aluminum content of the vaccines," *Pediatric Allergy an Immunology* 5, no. 2 (June 2007): 118–123.

43. Becker AB, et al. "Delay in diphtheria, pertussis, tetanus vaccination is associated with a reduced risk of childhood asthma, *J Allergy Clin Immunol*, No. 3 (March, 2008): 626-31.

44. T. Shirakawa et al., "The inverse association between tuberculin responses and atopic disorder," *Science* 275, no. 5296 (Jan. 1997): 77–79.

45. J. Li et al., "Absence of relationships between tuberculin responses and development of adult asthma with rhinitis and atopy," *Chest* 133 (2008): 100–106; R. Balicer et al., "Is childhood vaccination associated with asthma? A meta-analysis of observational studies," *Pediatrics* 120, no. 5 (Nov. 2007): 1269–1277.

46. E. Ostblom, et al., "Phenotypes of food hypersensitivity and development of allergic diseases during the first 8 years of life," *Clin Exp Allergy*, 38 (8) (2008): 1325-32.

47. Leon S. Kind, L. Roesner, "Enhanced susceptibility of pertussis inoculated mice to pollen extract," *Proc Soc Exp Biol Med*, 100, no. 4 (April 1959): 808–10.

48. C. Chang, R. Y. Gottshall, "Sensitization to ragweed pollen in Bordetella pertussis infected or vaccine-injected mice," *Journal of Allergy and Clinical Immunology*, 54, no. 1 (July 1974): 20–24.

49. R. Fischer et al., "Oral and nasal sensitization Promote distinct immune responses and reactivity in a mouse model of peanut allergy," *American Journal of Pathology*, 167 (2005): 1621–1630.

50. M. Profet, "The Function of Allergy," 26.

51. A. Mercae, *From immunology to social policy* (2003).

52. Cookson et al., "Asthma, An epidemic in the absence of infection?" *Science Magazine* 275, no. 5296 (Jan. 1997): 41–442.

53. M. Wjst, "The Triple T Allergy Hypothesis," *Clinical & Developmental Immunology* 11, no. 2 (June 2004): 175–80.

54. 44. M. Ryan et al., "Distinct T-cell subtypes induced with whole cell and acellular pertussis vaccines in children," *Immunology* 93 (1998): 1–10. Quoted in A. Mercae, *From immunology to social policy* 24.

55. D. Granoff, "Are serological responses to acellular pertussis antigens sufficient criteria to ensure that new combination vaccines are effective for prevention of

disease?" *Developments in Biological Standardisation* 89 (1997): 379–89. Quoted in A. Mercae, *From immunology to social policy* 24.

56. J. M. van Oosterhout, A. C. Motta, "Th1/Th2 paradigm: Not seeing the forest for the trees?" *European Respiratory Journal* 25 (2005): 591–593.

57. S. H. Sicherer et al., "US prevalence of self-reported peanut, tree nut, and sesame allergy: 11-year follow up," *J Allergy Clin Immunol* 125, 6 (June 2010): 1322–1326.

58. Ibid.

59. T. D. Green et al. "Clinical Characteristics of Peanut-Allergic Children: Recent Changes," *Pediatrics* 120, no. 6 (Dec. 2007): 1304–1310.

60. Ibid.

61. T. D. Green, "Clinical Characteristics of Peanut-Allergic Children," 8.

62. Ibid.

63. S. Sicherer et al. "Clinical features of acute allergic reactions to peanut and tree nuts in children," *Pediatrics* 102, no. 1 (1997).

64. T. Vander Leek et al., "The natural history of peanut allergy in young children and its association with serum peanut-specific IgE," *J Pediatr* 137 (2000): 749–755; and H. Skolnik et al., "The natural history of peanut allergy," *J Allergy Clin Immunol* 107 (2007): 367–374.

65. Mullins, Op. cit., 4.

66. S. Sicherer et al., "Prevalence of peanut and tree nut allergy in the United States determined by means of a random digit dial telephone survey: A 5 year follow up study." *Journal of Allergy and Clin Immunol* 112 (2003): 1203–1207.

67. M. D. Kogan et al., "Prevalence of parent-reported diagnosis of autism spectrum disorder among children in the U.S., 2007," *Pediatrics* (October 5, 2009).

68. C. J. Newschaffer et al., "National Autism Prevalence Trends from United States Special Education Data," *Pediatrics* 115, no. 3 (March 2005): 277–282.

69. Sex ratio, the proportion of male to female births, is indicative of reproductive health in all animals. A dramatic decline in male births in the Aamjiwnaang First Nation community between 1999 and 2003 startled researchers. Ratio of births in this period was about 33% boys and 67% girls, a ratio of 2:1. This community of 850 people resides on the St. Clair River near Sarnia, Ontario. It is believed that the trend is the result of exposures to endocrine-disrupting effluent and emissions of nearby petrochemical plants. The toxins include phthalates, a plasticizer to which humans are exposed daily in soft plastics, skin creams, shampoo, hair condition, and more.

70. R. Lockey, "Mechanisms of Anaphylaxis," *Life-Threatening Allergy, an Homage to Von Pirquet,* Mp3 lecture, World Allergy Forum, Vienna (June 11, 2006).

71. P. J. Hannaway et al., "Differences in race ethnicity, and socioeconomic status in school children dispensed injectable epinephrine in 3 Massachusetts school districts," *Ann Allergy Asthma Immunol* 95, no. 2 (Aug. 2005): 143–8.

72. C. Kuehni et al., "Food intolerance and wheezing in young South Asian and white children: Prevalence and clinical significance," *Journal of Allergy and Clinical Immunology* 118 (2006): 528–30; and F. Cataldo et al., "Are food intolerances and allergies increasing in immigrant children coming from developing countries?" *Pediatric Allergy and Immunology* 17 (2006): 364–69.

73. C. Kuehni, "Food intolerance and wheezing in young South Asian and white children," 528–30.

74. M. Eggesbo et al., "Is Delivery by Cesarean section a risk factor for food allergy?" *Journal of Allergy and Clinical Immunology* 112, no. 2 (2003): 420–426.

75. B. Laubereau et al., "Caesarean section and gastrointestinal symptoms, atopic dermatitis and sensitization during the first year of life," *Archives of Disease in Childhood* 89, no. 11 (Nov. 2004): 993–997.

76. M. Eggesbo, "Cesarean delivery and cowmilk allergy/intolerance," *Allergy* 60, no. 9 (Aug. 2005): 1172–73.

77. M. Kuitunen et al., "Probiotics prevent IgE associated allergy until age 5 years in cesarean-delivered children but not in the total cohort," *Journal of Allergy and Clinical Immunology* 10 (2008): 1016.

78. M. L. Moore, "Reducing the rate of Cesarean birth," *The Journal of Perinatal Education* 11, no. 2 (Spring 2002): 41–43.

79. J. A. Martin, "Births: Final data for 2006," *National Vital Statistics Reports, CDC* 57, no. 7.

80. A. Steinberg, *Encyclopedia of Jewish Medical Ethics* (Israel, Feldheim Publishers, 2003) 170.

81. R. Gonen, "Obstetricians' Opinions regarding patient choice in cesarean delivery," *Obstetrics & Gynecology* 99, no. 4 (April 2002): 577–580.

82. C. Weissman et al., "The Israeli anesthesiology physician workforce," *The Israel Medical Association Journal* 8 (April 2006).

83. I. Dalal et al., "Food allergy is a matter of geography after all: Sesame as a major cause of severe IgE mediated food allergic reactions among infants and young children in Israel," *Allergy* 57, no. 4 (April 2002): 362–5; and D. Aaronov et al., "Natural history of food allergy in infants and children in Israel," *Ann Allergy Asthma Immunol* 101, no. 6 (Dec. 2008): 637–40

84. J. O'B Hourihane, "The prevalence of peanut allergy in British children at school entry age in 2003," *Foodbase, Food Standards Agency* (May 31, 2006).

85. A. F. Dioun et al. "Is maternal age at delivery related to childhood food allergy? *Pediatr Allergy Immunol.* 14, no. 4 (Aug. 2003): 307–311.

86. www.allcountries.org/uscensus/90_cesarean_section_deliveries_by_age_ of.html.

87. Highlights from EAACI 2009, XXVIII Congress of he European Academy of Allergy and Clinical Immunology, June 6–10, Warsaw, Poland. www.

theucbinstituteofallergy.com/Images/EAACI_2009.pdf. Also, E. von Mutius et al., "Prevalence of asthma and atopy in two areas of West and East Germany," *American Journal of Respiratory and Critical Care Medicine* 149 (1994): 358–364.

88. D. Strachan, "Socioeconomic factors and the development of allergy," *Toxicology Letters* 86 (1996): 199–203.

89. C. Roehr et al., "Food allergy and non-allergic food hypersensitivity in children and adolescents," *Clinical & Experimental Allergy* 34, no. 1 (Oct. 2004): 1534–41.

90. A. Mehl et al., "Anaphylactic reactions in children—a questionnaire-based survey in Germany," *Allergy* 60, no. 11 (2005): 1440–1445.

91. A. Sheikh et al. "Anaphylaxis discharge rates by regional health authority, per 100,000 discharges," *Clin Exp Allergy* 31 (2001): 15671–76.

92. G. Lack et al., "Factors associated with the development of peanut allergy in childhood," *The New England Journal of Medicine* 348 (March 2003): 977–985.

93. M. P. Oryszczyn et al., "Head circumference at birth and maternal factors related to cord blood total IgE," *Clin Exp Allergy* 29, no. 3 (March 1999): 334–41.

94. V. Emerton (ed.), *Food allergy and intolerance: Current issues and concerns* (Great Britain, Royal Society of Chemistry, 2002) 11.

95. J. O'B Hourihane et al., "Peanut allergy in relation to heredity, maternal diet, and other atopic diseases: Results of a questionnaire survey, skin prick testing, and food challenges," *BMJ* 313 (1996): 518–521.

96. Ibid.

97. G. Lack et al., "Factors associated with the development of peanut allergy in childhood," *The New England Journal of Medicine* 348 (March 13, 2003): 977–985.

98. J. O'B. Hourihane, "Peanut allergy in relation to heredity, maternal diet, and other atopic diseases," 518–521.

99. S. Sicherer et al., "Genetics of peanut allergy: A twin study," *Journal of Allergy and Clinical Immunology* 106, no. 1 (July 2000): 53–56.

100. B. Bjorksten, "Genetic and Environmental Risk Factors for the Development of Food Allergy," *Current Opinion in Allergy and Clinical Immunology* 5, no. 3 (2005): 249–253.

101. Xiu-min Li et al., "Strain-dependent induction of allergic sensitization caused by peanut allergen DNA immunization in Mice," *The Journal of Immunology* 162 (1999): 3045–3052.

102. K. Bock, *Healing the New Childhood Epidemics.*

103. Ibid, 177.

104. Ibid, 51.

105. M. Hitti, "Childhood vaccination rates high," *Web MD Health News* (Sept. 4, 2008). http://children.webmd.com/vaccines/news/20080904/childhood-vaccination-rates-high.

106. Letter from Marlyn B. Maloney and Christopher H. Smith, Members of Congress in a letter to Hon. Kathleen Sebelius, Secretary, Health and Human Services, June 10, 2009.

107. Devi Lockwood, "Is there a link between vaccinations and peanut allergies," *Connecticut Science Fair* (2007) www.avoidingmilkprotein.com/vacandpea.htm.

108. Bock, *Healing the New Childhood Epidemics*, 57. Both Bock and Lockwood point out this CDC rationalization.

109. Vassileve, T.L., "Aluminum phosphate but not calcium phosphate stimulates the specific IgE response in guinea pigs to tetanus toxoid," *Allergy*, 33, No. 3 (June 1978): 155-9.

110. Love, B., 'Antibiotic exposure and the risk of food allergy in young children,' *JACI*, Vol. 131, No. 2 (Feb., 2013).

111. "Gut bacteria that protect against food allergies identified," Science Daily (Aug. 25, 2014).

112. Auinger, P., et al., "Trends in otitis media among children in the United States, *Pediatrics* 112 (2003):514–20.

113. Nsouli TM, et al., "Role of food allergy in serous otitis media," *Annals of Allergy*, 73(3), (Sept.,1994):215-9.

114. http://www.earallergy.com/ears-allergy/why-allergy-and-ear-disease/the-role-of-allergy/.

115. W. Leary, "Genetic engineering of crops can spread allergies, study shows," *New York Times* (March 14, 1996).

116. Liccardi, G., "Evaluation of the nocebo effect during oral challenge in patients with adverse drug reactions," *J Investig Allergol Clin Immunol*, 14 (2) (2004): 104-7.

117. Moseley, GL., et al., "The rubber hand illusion increases histamine reactivity in the real arm. Curr Biol. 6;21(23) (Dec. 2011).

118. H. Skolnick, et al., "The Natural history of peanut allergy," J Allergy Clin Immunol., 107 (2001): 367-374.

119. Ibid.

120. J. O'B. Hourihane et al., "Resolution of peanut allergy: Case-control study," *BMJ* 316 (1998): 1271–1275.

121. G. Du Toit et al., "Early consumption of peanuts in infancy is associated with a low prevalence of peanut allergy," *J Allergy Cli Immunol* 122 (Nov. 2008): 984–91; and G. Du Toit, "Learning Early about peanut allergy, The LEAP study," *The Newsletter of the British Society for Allergy & Clinical Immunology* 8 (Autumn, 2006): 6.

122. J. O'B Hourihane et al., "Resolution of peanut allergy following bone marrow transplantation for primary immunodeficiency," *Allergy* 60, no. 4 (April 2005): 536–537.

CHAPTER 3: THEORIES

1. L. Hammarstrom, C. Smith, "Immunologlobulin subclass distribution of specific antibodies in allergic patients," *Allergy* 42 (1987): 529–534.

2. www.nationaljewish.org/healthinfo/conditions/allergy/index.aspx National Jewish Health (August 2009); and J. Woodfolk, "Selective roles and dysregulation of interleukin-10 in allergic disease," *Current Allergy & Asthma Reports* 6, no. 1 (Jan. 2006): 40–46.

3. Reneé Dubos, *The Dreams of Reason: Science and Utopias* (New York, 1961) 71.

4. G. Lack et al. "Factors Associated with the Development of Peanut Allergy in Childhood," *The New England Journal of Medicine* 11, no. 348 (March 13, 2003): 977–985.

5. H. A. Sampson, "Peanut Allergy," *The New England Journal of Medicine* 346 (2002): 1294–1299.

6. R. Weeks, "Peanut oil in medications," *The Lancet* 348, no. 9029: 759–760. The World Standard Drug Database listed skin creams that contain peanut oil including: Calamine oily lotion, Eczederm cream, Hydromol cream, Hewletts cream, Kamillosan ointment, Masse cream, Siopel cream, zinc cream, Polytar emollient, and more.

7. Lack, "Factors Associated with the Development of Peanut Allergy in Childhood," 977–985.

8. J. Strid, J. O'B Hourihane et al., "Epicutaneous exposure to peanut protein prevents oral tolerance and enhances allergic sensitization," *Clin Exp.*, (June 2005).

9. Peeters et al., "Peanut allergy: Sensitization by peanut oil-containing local therapeutics seems unlikely," *J Allergy Clin Immunol* (May 2004).

10. L. O. McMurray, *George Washington Carver, Scientist & Symbol* (New York, Oxford University Press, 1981) 246.

11. Andrew Smith, *Peanuts, the Illustrious History of the Goober Pea* (Chicago, University of Illinois Press, 2002) 97.

12. U.S. FDA "Listing of Food Additive Status," (March 2009). See also www.cosmeticsdatabase.com/ingredient.php?ingred06=700482&nothanks=1.

13. A. Olszewski et al., "Isolation and characterization of proteic allergens in refined peanut oil," *Clin Exp Allergy* 28, no. 7 (July 1998): 850–9. "In conclusion, we have demonstrated the presence of allergenic proteins in crude and refined peanut oil. These proteins are the same size as two allergens previously described in peanut protein extracts." G. Lack et al., "Avon Longitudinal Study of Parents and Children Study Team. Factors associated with the development of peanut allergy in childhood," *N Engl J Med* 348 (2003): 977–85.

14. www.cfsan.fda.gov/~Dms/Alrgn.Html.

15. www.whc-oils.com/refined-peanut-oil.html.

16. The USP-NF is a book of public pharmacopeial standards containing standards for medicines, excipients, etc. In it is a "procedure" for refining peanut oil. www.usp.org/pdf/EN/monoRedesign/NF-Monos-I-Z.pdf.

17. J. B. Greig & Joint FAO/WHO Expert Committee on Food Additives, "Potential allergenicity of refined food products, peanut oils and soya bean oils," *WHO Food Additive Series, International Program on Chemical Safety*, 44 (2000): 8. www.inchem.org/documents/jecfa/jecmono/v44jec11.htm.

18. Ibid.

19. G. De Montis et al., "Sensitization to peanut and vitamin D oily preparations," *Lancet* 341 (1993): 1411.

20. D. A. Moneret-Vautrin et al., "Risk of milk formulas containing peanut oil contaminated with peanut allergens in infants with atopic dermatitis," *Pediatr Allergy Immunol* 5, no. 3 (Dec. 1993): 184–188.

21. A. Cantani, "Anaphylaxis from peanut oil in infant feedings and medications," *European Review of Medical and Pharmacological Sciences* 2 (1998): 203–206; and D. A. Moneret-Vautrin et al., "Risk of milk formulas containing peanut oil," 184–188.

22. "Refined Peanut Oil NF., FDA Registered, CGMP Proven Quality, All Natural," Welch, Holm & Clark Col, Inc. www.whc-oils.com/refined-peanut-oil.html.

23. S. Sicherer S., H. Sampson, "Peanut allergy: Emerging concepts and approaches for a apparent epidemic," *Journal of Allergy and Clinical Immunology* 120, no. 3 (Sept. 2007): 491–503.

24. S. H. Sicherer et al., "Prevalence of peanut and tree nut allergy in the United States determined by means of a random digit dial telephone survey: A 5-year follow up study," *J Allergy Clin Immunol* 112, no. 6 (Dec. 2003): 1203–1207.

25. J. Bernhisel-Broadbent, H. Sampson, "Cross-allergenicity in the legume botanical family in children with food hypersensitivity," *J Allergy Clin Immunol* 83 (1989): 435–40.

26. R. J. Dearman, I. Kimber, "Proteins as allergens: A toxicological perspective," *Food allergy and intolerance: Current issues and concerns* (Great Britain, Royal Society of Chemistry, 2002): 14 ff.

27. M. Frieri, B. Kettelhut (ed.), *Food Hypersensitivity and adverse reactions: a practical guide for diagnosis Clinical Allergy and Immunology* (CRC Press, 1999): 84; and S. D. Kelleher et al. "Functional Chicken Muscle Protein Isolates . . . ," *53rd Annual Reciprocal Meat Conference, American Meat Science Association* (2000). www.meatscience.org. Beef serum albumin and muscle protein (BSA and BGG) has a molecular weight of between 17 and 66 kDa; albumin in egg 45 kDa.

28. S. J. Maleki et al., "Structure of the Major Peanut Allergen Ara h 1 May Protect IgE-Binding Epitopes from Degradation," *J Immunol* 164, no. 11 (June 2000): 5844–9.

29. D. J. DeNoon, "CDC: 4% of U.S. Children New Suffer Food Allergies," MedicineNet.com (Oct. 22, 2008); and K. Beyer et al., "Effects of cooking methods on peanut allergenicity," *J Allergy Clin Immunol* 107 (2001): 1077–81.

30. M. Khodoun et al., "Peanuts can contribute to anaphylactic shock by activating complement," *J Allergy Clin Immunol* 123, no. 2 (Feb. 2009): 333–351.

31. S. J. Koppelman, "Quantification of major peanut allergens Ara h 1 and Ara h 2 in the peanut varieties Runner, Spanish, Virginia, and Valencia, bred in different parts of the world," *Allergy* 56, no. 2 (Feb. 2001): 132–7.

32. G. Du Toit et al., "Early consumption of peanuts in infancy is associated with a low prevalence of peanut allergy," *Journal of Allergy and Clinical Immunology* (November, 2008).

33. Charles Richet, *The Nobel Prize in Physiology or Medicine 1913, Nobel Lecture* (Dec. 11, 1913). http://nobelprize.org/nobel_prizes/medicine/laureates/1913/richet-lecture.html.

34. M. Profet, "The Function of Allergy: Immunological Defense Against Toxins," *The Quarterly Review of Biology* 66, no. 1 (1991).

35. Ibid., 38.

36. R. Fischer et al., "Oral and Nasal Sensitization Promote distinct immune responses and reactivity in a mouse model of peanut allergy," *American Journal of Pathology* 167 (2005): 1621–1630; and F. van Wijk et al., "The CD28/CTLA-4-B7 signaling pathway is involved in both allergic sensitization ad tolerance induction to orally administered peanut proteins," *The Journal of Immunology* 178 (2007): 6894–6900.

37. J. W. Coleman, M. Blanca, "Mechanisms of drug allergy," *Immunology Today* 19, no. 5 (May 1998): 196–198; A. Cantani, *Pediatric allergy, asthma and immunology* (Germany, Springer, 2008): 1150; and A. L. Schocket (ed.), *Clinical management of uticaria and anaphylaxis* (U.S., Marcel Dekker, Inc., 1993): 120.

38. M. Frieri, B. Kettelhut, *Food hypersensitivity and adverse reactions: A practical guide for diagnosis* (CRC Press, 1999): 81.

39. A. Cantani, *Pediatric allergy, asthma and immunology*, 214.

40. Profet, "The Function of Allergy," 35.

41. Ibid, 36.

42. O. L. Frick, D. L. Brooks, "Immunologloglubulin E antibodies to pollens augmented in dogs by virus vaccines," *Am. J. Vet. Res* 44 (1983): 440–445. Quoted in Profet, "The Function of Allergy," 46.

43. N. R. Lynch, et al., "Allergic reactivity and helminthic infection in Amerindians of the Amazon Basin," *Int Arch Allergy Appl Immunol* 72 (1983): 369–72.

44. S. Scrivener et al. "Independent effects of intestinal parasite infection and domestic allergen exposure on risk of wheeze in Ethiopia: A case-control study," *Lancet* 358 (2001): 1493–1499.

45. A. H. Van den Biggelaar et al., "The prevalence of parasite infestation and house dust mite sensitization in Gabonese schoolchildren," *Int Arch Allergy Immunol* 126 (2001): 231–238.

46. D. E. Elliot et al., "Helminths as governors of immune-mediated inflammation," *International Journal for Parasitology* (2007).

47. R. M. Maizels, M. Yazdanbakhsh, "Immune regulation by helminth parasites: cellular and molecular mechanisms," *Nature Reviews, Immunology* 3 (Sept. 2003): 733.

48. E. A. Sabin et al. "Impairment of tetanus toxoid-specific Th1-like immune responses in humans infected with Schistosoma mansoni," *J Infect. Dis* 173 (1996): 269–272; and A. J. Macdonald et al. "A novel, helminth-derived immuostimulant enhances human recall response to hepatitis C virus and tetanus toxoid and is dependent on CD56+ cells for its action," *Clin Exp Immunol* 152 (2008): 265–273.

49. Klaus Erb, "Can helminths or helminth-derived products be used in humans to prevent or treat allergic diseases?" *Trends in Immunology* 30, no. 2 (Feb. 2009): 75–82.

50. M. Yazdanbakhsh, S. Wahyuni, "The role of helminth infections in protection from atopic disorders," *Current Opinion in Allergy and Clinical Immunology* 5 (2005): 386–391.

51. Ibid.

52. K. J. Erb, "Helminths, allergic disorders and IgE-mediated immune responses: where do we stand?" *European Journal of Immunology* 37, no. 5 (April 2007): 1170–1173.

53. Ibid.

54. Profet, "The Function of Allergy," 48.

55. B. Ogilivie, V. Jones. "Immunity in the parasitic relationships between helminths and hosts," *Progress in Allergy* 17 (1973): 93–144; and M. L. Baeza et al. "Anisakis simplex allergy: a murine model of anaphylaxis induced by parasitic proteins displays a mixed Th1Thx pattern," *British Society for Immunology* 142, no. 3 (Dec. 2005): 433–440.

56. D. A. Johnson, "Is H. Pylori infection protective against asthma and allergies?" *Gastroenterology* 57 (May 2008): 561; and Y. Chen, M. J. Blaser, "Inverse associations of Helicobacter pylori with asthma and allergy," *Archives of Internal Medicine* 167 (2007): 821–827.

57. P. G. Engelkirk, *Laboratory diagnosis of infectious diseases* (Philadelphia, Wolters Kluwer Health, 2008): 596.

58. B. E. Zacharia, P. Sherman, "Allergies, helminths, and cancer," *Medical Hypotheses* 60 (Sept. 2005): 1–5.

59. A. Gosline, "Peanut allergy: dining with death," *New Scientist* 2557 (June 21, 2006). www.newscientist.com/article/mg19025571.500-peanut-allergy- dining-with-death.html?page=3.

60. L. Chiu et al. "Estimation of the sensitization rate to peanut by prick skin test in the general population: results from the National Health and Nutrition Examination Survey, 1980–1994," *J Allergy Clin Immunol* 107 (2001): S192.

61. "Current Trends in Allergic Reactions: a multidisciplinary approach t patient management," *Clinician, National Institute of Allergy and Infectious diseases of the National Institutes of Health, US Dept. of Health and Human Services* 21, no. 3 (Sept. 2003).

62. D. P. Strachan, "Family size, infection and atopy: the first decade of the hygiene hypothesis," *Thorax* 55 (2000): S2–S10.

63. K. L. McDonald et al., "Delay in diphtheria, pertussis, tetanus vaccination is associated with a reduced risk of childhood asthma," *J Allergy Clin Immuol* 121, no. 3 (March 2008): 626–631.

64. Ibid., S8.

65. M. Akdis et al. "T regulatory cells in allergy: novel concepts in the pathogenesis, prevention and treatment of allergic diseases," *J Allergy Clin Immuol* 116, no. 5 (Nov. 2005): 961–8.

66. Profet, Op. cit., 46.

67. O. L. Frick, D. L. Brooks, "Immunolglobulin E antibodies to pollens augmented in dogs by virus vaccines," *Am. J. Vet. Res* 44 (1983): 440–445. Quoted in Profet, Op. cit., 46.

68. C. Chang, R. Y. Gottshall, "Sensitization to ragweed pollen in Bordetella pertussis-infected or vaccine-injected mice," *J Allergy Clin Immuol* 54, no. 1 (July 1974): 20–24.

69. M. Yazdanbakhsh, "The role of helminth infections in protection from atopic disorders," 386–391.

70. J. Diamond, "The Worst Mistake in the History of the Human Race," *Discover Magazine* (May 1987). See also J. Diamond, *Guns, Germs and Steel* (2005).

71. "Gut bacteria that protect against food allergies identified," Science Daily (Aug. 25, 2014).

72. Love, B., 'Antibiotic exposure and the risk of food allergy in young children,' *JACI*, Vol. 131, No. 2 (Feb., 2013).

73. Auinger, P. et al., "Trends in otitis media among children in the United States," *Pediatrics* (2003)112:514–20)

74. Nsouli TM, et al., "Role of food allergy in serous otitis media," *Annals of Allergy*, 73(3), (Sept.,1994):215-9.

75. http://www.earallergy.com/ears-allergy/why-allergy-and-ear-disease/the-role-of-allergy/.

76. http://www.foxnews.com/health/2012/09/12/peanut-allergies-seen-on-rise/#ixzz26MCWhtqZ

CHAPTER 4: REDISCOVERING ANAPHYLAXIS

1. J. Ring, H. Behrendt, "Anaphylaxis and Anaphylactoid Reactions," *Clinical Reviews in Allergy and Immunology* 7, no. 4 (Dec. 1999).

2. L. H. Freude, J. Rejaunier, *The Complete Idiot's Guide to Food Allergies* (New York: Penguin Group, 2003): 14.

3. Mark Jackson, *Allergy, The History of a Modern Malady* (London: Reaktion Books, 2007): 28.

4. Jared Diamond, "The Worst Mistake in the History of the Human Race," *Discover Magazine* (May 1987).

5. Ibid.

6. Richard Preston, *The Demon in the Freezer, a true story* (New York: Random House, 2002): 24.

7. S. Riedel, "Edward Jenner and the history of smallpox and vaccination," *Proceedings (Bayl Univ Med Cent)* 18, no. 1 (Jan. 2005): 21–25.

8. Edward Jenner, *An inquiry into the causes and effects of the variolae vaccinae* (London, 1798).

9. J. G. Rigau-Perez, "The Introduction of Smallpox Vaccine in 1803 and the Adoption of Immunization as a Government Function in Puerto Rico," *Hispanic American Historical Review* 69, no. 3 (1989): 393–423, quoted in A. Minna Stern, H. Markel, "The History of Vaccines and Immunization: Familiar Patterns, New Challenges," *Health Affairs* 24, no. 3 (2005): 611–621.

10. H. Davies, "Ethical reflections on Edward Jenner's experimental treatment," *Journal of Medical Ethics* 33 (2007): 174–176. The inoculation technique was developed in China, Africa, and India well before the eighteenth century when English aristocrat Lady Mary Wortley Montague introduced it to Europe. Lady Mary's brother had died of smallpox, and she herself had suffered an episode that disfigured her face. Convinced that inoculation was the lesser of two evils, she had both her children treated. Subsequent inoculations of prisoners and orphans were deemed a success when no one died. Ultimately in 1722, the two daughters of the Princess of

Wales were inoculated without incident. With this star endorsement, the technique began to gain acceptance.

11. D. Baxby, "Smallpox vaccination techniques; from knives and forks to needles and pins," *Vaccine* 20, no. 16 (May 2002): 2140–2149.

12. A. B. Steele, "Vaccination at Shorncliffe," *Lancet* 76, no. 1923 (July 1860): 46.

13. D. A. Henderson, "Edward Jenner's vaccine," *Public Health Reports* (Mar/April 1997): 112.

14. J. B. Tucker, *Scourge: The Once and Future Threat of Smallpox* (New York: Atlantic Monthly Press, 2001).

15. T. Reimer, *Smallpox and Vaccination in the Civil War: National Museum of Civil War Medicine* (NMCWM Press, 2004). http:www.civilwarmed.org.

16. I. Berry, R. Martin, *The Pharmaceutical Regulatory Process* (Informa Health care, 2008): 6.

17. R. Porter, *Disease, Medicine and Society in England, 1550–1860* (Cambridge U. Press, 1995): 42.

18. P. W. Laird, *Advertising progress: American business and the rise of consumer marketing* (Baltimore: Johns Hopkins University Press 1998): 480. Quoted in Kalman Applbaum "Pharmaceutical Marketing and the Invention of the Medical Consumer," *PLoS Med (Public Library of Science)* 3, no. 4 (April 2006).

19. David Lilienfeld, "The First Pharmacoepidemiologic Investigations national drug safety policy in the United States, 1901–1902," *Perspectives in Biology and Medicine* 51, no. 2 (Spring 2008). Renowned psychiatrist Sigmund Freud quoted articles from this publication and made financial arrangements with Parke, Davis, and Merck to support research in *On Coca* (1884). In this publication he supported the beneficial effects of cocaine for many problems including morphine addiction.

20. Ibid.

21. L. Glambos, J. Eliot Sewell, *Networks of Innovation: Vaccine Development at Merck, Sharp and Dohme, and Mulford, 1895–1995* (New York: Cambridge U. Press, 1995). When Mulford went into decline in the 1920s it was purchased in 1929 by Sharp & Dohme. This company merged with Merck in 1953. Merck dominated the marketplace in 2009.

22. Anne Hardy, *The Epidemic Streets: infectious disease and the rise of preventive medicine, 1856–1900* (Oxford U. Press, 1993): 83.

23. William Bynum, *Science and the Practice of Medicine in the Nineteenth Century* (Cambridge University Press, 1994): 164.

24. Ibid., 161.

25. "Horse 397, Condemned as useless, proved worth $175,000," *The New York Times* (June 7, 1914).

26. F. J. Grunbacher. "Behring's discovery of Dip and tetanus antitoxins," *Immunology Today* 13 (1992): 188–90. Quoted in Jackson, Op. cit., 31.

27. R. A. Kondratas, "Biologics Control Act of 1902," *The Early Years of Federal Food and Drug Control* (1982): 8–27. Quoted in Lilienfeld, Op. cit.

28. I. Berry, R. Martin, *The Pharmaceutical Regulatory Process* (Informa Health care, 2008): 3.

29. Ibid., 5.

30. "Attorney General Acts Against Drug Trust, Seeks an Injunction to Prevent Control of Prices, Suit Brought in Indiana, Proprietary and Wholesale and Retail Druggists' Associations Named as Defendants, Conspiracy Charged," *The New York Times* (May 10, 1906).

31. Stuart Anderson, *Making Medicines: A brief history of pharmacy and pharmaceuticals* (Pharmaceutical Press, 2005): 156.

32. Intravenous injection and infusion began as early as 1670.

33. Gary Matsumoto, *Vaccine A* (Basic Books, 2004): 26.

34. K. Stratton et al., *Adverse Events Associated with Childhood Vaccines* (National Academies Press, 1994): 223–224.

35. E. A. Belongia, A. L. Naleway, "Smallpox Vaccine: The Good, the Bad and the Ugly," *Clinical Medicine & Research* 1, no. 2 (April 2003): 87–92. The authors of this article attempt to show that the "vaccine is a critical tool for controlling smallpox ("the good"), despite a relatively higher risk of complications in some individuals ("the bad"). The "ugly" refers not to the vaccine, but to the potential reintroduction of smallpox more than twenty years after its eradication." M. Hassani et al., "Vaccines for the prevention of diseases caused by potential bioweapons," *Clinical Immunology* 111, no. 1 (April 2004): 1–15.

36. Vaughan, *Strange Malady*, 46.

37. A. Nelson, C. Horsburgh, *Pathology of Emerging Infections 2* (ASM Press, 1998), 146.

38. M. Meddow Bayly, "Some Little-Understood Effects of Serum Therapy," *Medical World* (April 6, 1934).

39. Clemens von Pirquet, "On the Theory of Infectious Diseases" (April 1903). Cited by Jackson, *Allergy*: 35–36.

40. C. Von Pirquet, B. Schick, *Serum Sickness* (1905). Translated by B. Schick (Baltimore, 1951).

41. C. Von Pirquet, "Allergie," *Munchener Medizinische Wochenschrift* (1906). Cited in Jackson, *Allergy*: 37.

42. Vaughan, *Strange Malady*: 46.

43. Nadja Durbach, *Bodily Matters: The Anti-vaccination Movement in England, 1853– 1907* (Durham: Duke University Press, 2005): 97.

44. Ibid., 100.

45.   G. T. Keusch, "The History of nutrition: Malnutrition, infection and immunity," *Journal of Nutrition* 133, no.1 (Jan. 2003): 336S–340S. It is less well publicized that Western nutrition science grew concurrent with biomedical research. Knowledge of host nutritional status and immunity was well established. Food as a cure or prevention for disease was a concept explored by Hippocrates in 400 BC who encouraged his students to "let thy food be thy medicine." The term "vitamins" was coined by Dr. Casmir Funk in 1912. In 1930, William Rose discovered essential amino acids, building blocks of proteins. The cyclical relationship between poor nutrition or malnutrition such as the severe "kwashiorkor" resulting from insufficient dietary protein and the spread of infectious disease was not well documented before 1959. Eleanora McBean, *The Poisoned Needle* (Health Research Books, 1957, 1993) 10. www.scribd.com/doc/12983463/The-Poisoned- Needle-by-Eleanor-Mcbean.

46.   George Bernard Shaw, "Preface," *Doctor's Dilemma* (1909).

47.   Richet, *The Nobel Prize in Physiology or Medicine 1913, Nobel Lecture* (Dec. 11, 1913).

48.   Ibid.

49.   Ibid.

50.   Richet noticed that anaphylactized animals even when they seem in perfect health have leucocytes that often exceed two hundred.

51.   A. Besredka, P Roux, *Anaphylaxis and Anti-Anaphylaxis* (London, Heinemann, 1919): 18.

52.   Richet, *Nobel Lecture*.

53.   Ibid.

54.   Vaughan, *Strange Malady*: 110.

55.   Ilana Lowy, "On guinea pigs, dogs and men: Anaphylaxis and the study of biological individuality, 1902–1939," *Studies in History and Philosophy of Science Part C* 34, no. 3 (Sept. 2003): 399–423.

56.   A. Schofield, "A Case of Egg Poisoning," *Lancet* (1908): 716.

57.   O. Schloss, "A Case of Allergy to Common Foods," *American Journal of Diseases of Children* 3 (1912): 341.

58.   J. Hettwer, R. Kriz, "Absorption of Undigested Protein from the Alimentary Tract as Determined by the Direct Anaphylaxis Test," *American Journal of Physiology* 73 (1925): 539–546.

59.   Clinical allergy focused on environment allergies and desensitization through injection. British allergists John Freeman and Leonard Noon published accounts of injecting increasing doses of an extract of pollen to reduce sensitivity to same in 1911. Others experimented with desensitization: B. Keston et al., "Oral Desensitization to Common Foods," *J Allergy*, 6 (1935): 431; and T. G. Randolph,

"Allergy as a Causative Factor of Fatigue, Irritability, and Behavioral Problems of Children," *J Pediatrics* 31 (1947): 560–572.

60. W. T. Longcope, F. M. Rachemann, "Severe renal insufficiency associated with attacks of urticaria in hypersensitive individuals," *Journal of Urology* 1 (1917): 351; W. Duke, "Food allergy as a cause of abdominal pain," *Arch Int Med*, 28 (1921): 151; W. Duke, "Food allergy as a cause of bladder pain," *Ann Clin Med.*, 1, (1922): 117; and W.Duke, "Meniere's syndrome caused by allergies," *JAMA* 81 (1923): 2179.

61. Vaughan, *Strange Malady*: 109.

62. S. Plotkin et al., *Vaccines* (Elsevier Health Sciences, 2008): 6.

63. Vaughan, 46.

64. A. Besredka, *Anaphylaxis and Anti-Anaphylaxis and Their Experimental Foundations* (London: William Henkmann (Medical Books Ltd., 1919).

65. H. M. Gezon et al., "A new repository penicillin (a form of aqueous penicillin G procaine) in infants and children," *Pediatrics* 4 (July 1949): 15; A. B. Cannon et al., "Maintenance of penicillin blood levels after a single intramuscular injection of penicillin in various oils," *Science* 104, no. 2705 (Nov. 1946): 414–415; and W. G. Myers, "The urinary excretion of penicillin after ingestion with and without adjuvants and following intramuscular injection," *The Ohio Journal of Science* 46, no. 2 (March 1946): 53–64. https://kb.osu.edu/dspace/bitstream/1811/3508/1/V46N02_053.pdf.

66. "Products and Processes," *Chemical and Engineering News* 23, no. 5 (March 1945): 466–468.

67. Judy Hankins, *Infusion Therapy in Clinical Practice* (Elsivier, 2001): 3.

68. Francoise Nielloud, Gilberte Marti-Mestres, *Pharmaceutical emulsions and suspensions* (CRC Press, 2000): 236.

69. E. J. Coulson, J. R. Spies, "The Immunochemistry of allergens III, Anaphylactogenic potenticy of the electrophoretic fractionation products of CS-1A from Cottonseed," *The Journal of Immunology* 46 (1943): 367–376.

70. Vaughan, *Strange Malady*: 155.

71. Earlier articles in literature cited in F. M. Atkins et al., "Cottonseed hypersensitivity: new concerns over an old problem," *J Allergy Clin Immunol* 82, no. 2 (Aug. 1988): 242–50; and T. G. Randolph, "Cottonseed protein vs. cottonseed oil sensitivity; a case of cottonseed oil sensitivity," *Ann Allergy* 8, no. 1 (Jan.–Feb. 1950): 5–10.

72. National Cottonseed Products Association and the U.S. Federal Security Agency, *Allergy to cottonseed and other oilseeds and their edible derivatives. Excerpts from testimony before the Administrator, Federal Security Agency in the matter of fixing and establishing definitions and standards of identity for mayonnaise, French dressing, and related salad dressings (Docket FDC-51) Public hearings held at*

Washington DC, Nov. 18, 1947, and January 6 to 8, 1948 (Memphis, National Cottonseed Products Assn., 1948).

73. "Allergy to cottonseed and other oil seeds and the edible derivatives," *California Medicine* 71, no. 5 (Nov. 1949): 384.

74. Garry Nall, "Encyclopedia of Oklahoma history & culture," *Oklahoma Historical Society* (undated). http://digital.library.okstate.edu/encyclopedia/entries/C/CO066.html.

75. Lynette Boney Wrenn, *Cinderella of the New South: A History of the Cottonseed Industry, 1855–1955* (Knoxville, University of Tennessee Press, 1995).

76. Based on online review of medical journals as well as information in F. M. Atkins et al., "Cottonseed hypersensitivity: new concerns over an old problem," *J Allergy Clin Immunol* 82, no. 2 (Aug. 1988): 242–50.

77. Website of Welch Holme Clark, www.welch-holme-clark.com/peanut_oil_-_refined_spec_-_ve.html.

78. F. W. Denny et al., "Comparative effects of penicillin, auremycin and terramycin on streptococcal tonsillitis and pharyngitis," *Pediatrics* 11 (Jan. 1953): 7–14.

CHAPTER 5: THE HISTORY OF PEANUT ALLERGY

1. The story of Patricia Malone, published in the *NY Journal American* won a Pulitzer Prize in 1944.

2. David Wilson, *In Search of Penicillin* (Knopf, 1976); and David Greenwood, *Antimicrobial Drugs, Chronicle of a Twentieth Century Medical Triumph* (Oxford University Press, 2008) 120. Through the 1940s, efforts to produce the same wonder drug in Germany, Ausria, Czechoslovakia, and other countries had yielded results but were delayed with the end of World War II.

3. Monroe J. Romansky, George E. Rittman, "A method of prolonging the action of penicillin," *Science* 100, no. 2592 (Sept. 1 1944): 196–198.

4. T. Guthe et al., "Untoward penicillin reactions," *Bulletin, World Health Organization* 19, no. 3 (1958): 427–501.

5. Francis H. Chafee, "Sensitivity to peanut oil with the report of a case," *Annals of Internal Medicine* 15, no. 6 (Dec. 1, 1941): 1116–1117.

6. P. C. Trussell et al., "Duration of Effective Blood levels following administration of penicillin in peanut oil and beeswax," *Canadian Medical Association Journal* 57 (Oct. 1947): 387; R. V. Platou et al., "Round Table Discussion on Antibiotics," *Pediatrics* 1 (Feb. 1948): 270–287; and B. M. Kagan et al., "Studies of Penicillin in Pediatrics: III, Procaine Penicillin G in Sesame Oil, in Peanut Oil with 2%

Aluminum Monostearate and in Water with Sodium Carboxmethylcellulose," *Pediatrics* 5, no. 4 (April 1950): 664–671.

7. G. Hildick-Smith et al., "Penicillin Regimens in Pediatric Practice: Study of Blood Levels," *Pediatrics* (Jan. 1950): 97–113.

8. T. E. Roy, Antibiotics and iatrogenic disease," *Pediatrics* 22 (1958); 167.

9. Guthe, "Untoward penicillin reactions," (1958); and Kagan, "Studies of Penicillin and Pediatrics" (1950).

10. Guthe, "Untoward pencillin reactions" (1958): 451.

11. Kagan, "Studies of Penicillin and Pediatrics" (1950).

12. J. M. Bond et al. "The second international reference preparation of procaine benzylpenicillin in oil with aluminum monostearate," *Bulletin of the World Health Organization* 48, no. 1 (1973): 91–8; and R. R. Willcox, "Treatment of syphilis," *Bulletin of the World Health Organization* 59, no. 5 (1981): 655–663.

13. Guthe, "Untoward penicillin reactions" (1958).

14. "Doctors warn of increasing penicillin peril, some are susceptible to shock, death," *Chicago Daily Tribune* (May 8, 1953): 22.

15. V. A. Drill, *Pharmacology in Medicine: A Collaborative Textbook* (New York, Toronto, London): 1954. Quoted by Guthe, "Untoward penicillin reactions" (1958).

16. A. Olszewski et al., "Isolation and characterization of proteic allergens in refined peanut oil," *Clin Exp Allergy* 28, no. 7 (July 1998): 850–9. "In conclusion, we have demonstrated the presence of allergenic proteins in crude and refined peanut oil. These proteins are the same size as two allergens previously described in peanut protein extracts."

17. The Threshold Working Group, *Approaches to establish thresholds for major food allergens and for gluten in food* (FDA, March 2006). www.fda.gov/Food/LabelingNutrition/FoodAllergensLabeling/GuidanceComplianceRegulatory Information/ucm106108.htm.

18. J. B. Greig & Joint FAO/WHO Expert Committee on Food Additives, "Potential allergenicity of refined food products, peanut oils and soya bean oils," *WHO Food Additive Series: 44* (Geneva, WHO, International Program on Chemical Safety, 2000): 8. www.inchem.org/documents/jecfa/jecmono/v44jec11.htm.

19. D. A. Moneret-Vautrin et al., "Risk of milk formulas containing peanut oil contaminated with peanut allergens in infants with atopic dermatitis," *Pediatr Allergy Immunol* 5, no. 3 (1994): 184–188; and G. De Montis et al., "Sensitization to peanut and vitamin D oily preparations," *Lancet* 341 (1993): 1411.

20. S. Sicherer et al., "U.S. prevalence of self-reported peanut, tree nut, and sesame allergy: 11-year follow-up," *The Journal of Allergy and Clinical Immunology* 125, no. 6 (June 2010): 1322–1326.

21. U.S. Patent 3,696,189, Oct. 3, 1972; and O. Kayser, H. Rainer, *Pharmaceutical biotechnology*, (Wiley-VCH, 2004) 27; A. E. Humphrey, F. H. Deindoerfer, "Microbiological Process Report," *Fermentation Process Review* (1960): 369. http://aem.asm.org/cgi/reprint/10/4/359.pdf.

22. F. Scott Smyth, "Asthma in Children, Round Table Discussion" *Pediatrics* 2, no. 1 (July 1948): 119–131.

23. R. C. Harris, "The Treatment of Tetanus: Report of Two Cases with Critical Comment on New Therapeutic Resources," *Pediatrics* 2 (Aug. 1948): 175–185.

24. A. Cantani, "Anaphylaxis from peanut oil in infant feedings and medications," *European Review of Medical and Pharmacological Sciences* 2 (1998): 203–206.

25. D. A. Moneret-Vautrin, "Risk of milk formulas containing peanut oil," 184–188.

26. Andrew Smith, *Peanuts, the illustrious history of the goober pea*, 65.

27. Ibid., 20.

28. Ibid., 67.

29. J. D. Stuart, "Peanuts and Patriotism," *Forum* 58 (Sept. 1917): 375–80. In Smith, *Peanuts*, 205.

30. Smith, *Peanuts*, 100.

31. CDC, *National Occupational Exposure Survey (1981–1983)*. At greatest risk for hazardous exposure to peanut oil in the early '80s were veterinarians closely followed by telephone installers and repairers. www.cdc.gov/noes/noes2/a1216occ.html.

32. Smith, *Peanuts*, 93.

33. Ibid., 102.

34. Ibid., 104.

35. Jane Holt, "News of Food; Peanut Crop, Worth $200,000,000 to South, Moving to Retail Stores in Various Forms," *The New York Times* (Sat., Nov. 11, 1944): 16.

36. Henry Lesesne, "Peanut Industry is Seeking Substitutes for War Uses, Report from the South," *St. Petersburg Times, Florida* (Sept. 24, 1945): 2.

37. Jane Holt, "News of Food; Latest Shortage Looms in Peanut Supply for Civilians With a 50% Cut Forecast," *The New York Times* (Sat. Jan. 6, 1945): 14.

38. Alfred Stefferud, "Big business in a nutshell," *New York Times Sunday Magazine* (Nov. 9, 1947): SM39.

39. Smith, *Peanuts*,104. "$10,000,000 worth of peanuts were sold last year by Mssrs. Obici and Peruzzi, who own Planters Nut and Chocolate Co.," *Fortune* (April 1938): 80. Quoted by Smith, *Peanuts*, 55.

40. R. B. Borges, "Trade and the political economy of agricultural policy: the case of the United States Peanut Program," *Journal of Agriculture and Applied Economics* 27, no. 2 (Dec. 1995): 595–612. http://ageconsearch.umn.edu/bitstream/15267/1/27020595.pdf. The Agricultural Act of 1949 established acreage allotments

for peanuts thus limiting the total amount of peanuts produced. Prior to 1978, all peanuts from these allotments were guaranteed a support price. These were quota peanuts. With technology more was grown on less land. For example, in 1950 allotment was 2,200,000 acres producing 2 billion pounds of peanuts. In 1981 allotment was 1,739 and production was nearly 4 billion pounds. Additional surplus quota peanuts were allowed, but certain rules and different prices apply.

41.   A. P. Black, "A new diagnostic method in allergic disease," *Pediatrics* 17 (May 1956): 716–724. S. Goldman et al., "Milk Allergy," *Pediatrics* 32 (Sept. 1963): 425–443; and W. G. Crook et al., "Systemic Manifestations due to allergy: Report on Fifty Patients," *Pediatrics* 27 (May 1961): 790–799. Both articles observe an increase in peanut and food allergy in children.

42.   Smith, *Peanuts*, 208.

43.   Borges, "Trade and the political economy of agricultural policy" (1995). NAFTA (1994), GATT (1995) and the U.S.-Canada Free Trade Agreement (1989) have complicated the market and threatened to remove import barriers. These fears were unfounded since the 1995 Farm Bill continued subsidy for the farmers.

44.   S. M. Fletcher, "Snack Peanuts Purchase Pattern," *Journal of Agricultural and Applied Economics* 34, no. 1 (April 2002).

45.   E. Foko, *Transforming Mature Industries into Growth Industries: The Case of US Peanuts* (Kansas State U., 2008, master of Agribusiness): 10.

46.   Stacy V. Jones, "Peanut Oil used in New Vaccine; product patented for Merck Said to Extend Immunity," *The New York Times, Business Financial Section* (Sept. 19, 1964): 31. Found online: http://pqasb.pqarchiver.com/djreprints/access/103910879.html?dids=103910879:103910879&FMT=ABS&FMTS=ABS:AI&type=historic&date=Nov+19%2C+1964&author=&pub=Wall+Street+Journal&desc=Merck+Says+Emulsion+Of+Peanut+Oil+Extends+Longevity+of+Flu+Shot&pqatl=google. Also reported in "Longer Life Vaccines," *The Age* (Australia, Monday, Dec. 7, 1964): 9.

47.   United States Patent Office, 3,149,036, Sept. 15, 1964.

48.   U.S. Patent 3,149,036, Sept. 15, 1964.

49.   Stacy V. Jones, "Peanut Oil used in New Vaccine" (1964).

50.   "Peanut Oil Additive Is Found to Improve Flu Shot's Potency," *New York Times* (Nov. 11, 1966): 33.

51.   Emulsifying A process for preparing a highly stable water-in-oil type emulsion consisting of a) a disperse aqueous phase; b) a continuous oil phase containing isomannide monooleate emulsifier and a nonhydrated physiologically acceptable fatty acid metal salt. A particular use of the invention is the preparation of an emulsion adjuvant vaccine, wherein the vaccine is incorporated in the aqueous phase. The emulsion is prepared by mixing the aqueous and oil phases at a relatively

low agitator speed, optionally cooling, increasing the speed of agitation to form an emulsion and optionally homogenizing the emulsion.

52. R. W. Howell, A. B. Mackenzie, "A Comparative trial of oil-adjuvant and aqueous polyvalent influencza vaccines," *British Journal of Industrial Medicine* 21 (1964): 265.

53. H. Nelson, "Expert Raises hope for improved flu vaccine, new serum produces 64 times more antibodies in animal tests, doctor says," *The Los Angeles Times* (April 14, 1969): A 25.

54. J. W. G. Smith et al., "Response to influenza vaccine in adjuvant 65-4," *Journal of Hygiene* 74, no. 2 (April 1974): 251–259; M. R. Hilleman, A. F. Woodhour AF, A. Friedman, A. H. Phelps, "Studies for safety of Adjuvant 65," *Ann. Allergy* 30 (1972): 477–80; and R. E. Weibel, A. McLean, A. F. Woodhour, A. Friedman, M. R. Hilleman, "Ten-year follow-up study for safety of Adjuvant 65 influenza vaccine in man," *Proceedings of the Society for Experimental Biology and Medicine* 143 (1973): 1053–6.

55. Hilleman supported the use of peanut oil adjuvant in other vaccines such as one for cancer. Quoted in R. Kotulak, "He wants to vaccinate your child against cancer," *Chicago Tribune* (Feb. 24, 1974): M24.

56. N. Petrovsky, J. Cesar Aguilar, "Vaccine Adjuvants: Current State and Future Trends," *Immunology and Cell Biology* 82 (2004): 488–496.

57. M. R. Hilleman et al., "Immunological Adjuvants, Report of a WHO Scientific Group," *World Health Organization Technical Report Series, no. 595* (Geneva, World Health Organisation, 1976): 9.

58. Ibid, 11.

59. The Threshold Working Group, *Approaches to establish thresholds for major food allergens and for gluten in food* (FDA, March 2006).

60. Derek Hobson, "The potential role of immunological adjuvants in influenza vaccines," *Postgraduate Medical Journal* 49 (March 1973): 180–184.

61. Ibid., 183.

62. Interview with Adjuvant 65 developer Dr. Maurice Hilleman in "Human Cancer Virus Vaccines," *Cancer Journal for Clinicians* 24 (1974): 212–217.

63. L. Galambos, *Networks of Innovation, Vaccine Development at Merck, Sharp & Dohme, and Mulford, 1895–1995* (Cambridge University Press, 1995): 138. The original Adjuvant 65 (1964) U.S. Pat. No. 3,149,036 was followed by U.S. Pat. No. 3,983,228 published Sept. 28, 1976 and U.S. Pat. No. 4,069,313 published in1978. Inventors of both adjuvants were A. F. Woodhour and M. R. Hilleman with the patent assigned to Merck & Co. Inc. The 1978 adjuvant for influenza improved on the original Adjuvant 65 (3149036 patent) in that it could be used with

"proteinaceous antigen." It had a longer shelf life and it used "pure materials" that withstood deemulsification.

64. Galambos, *Networks of Innovation*, 138.

65. Manmohan Singh (ed.), *Vaccine adjuvants and delivery systems* (New Jersey, Wiley, 2007): 6.

66. N. Goto et al., "Studies on the Toxicities of Aluminum Hydroxide and Calcium Phosphate as Immunological Adjuvants for Vaccines," *Vaccine* 11 (1993): 914–918; N. R. Butler et al., "Advantages of aluminum hydroxide adsorbed combined diphtheria, tetanus, and pertussis vaccines for the immunization of infants," *British Medical Journal* 1 1969): 663–666; F. M. Audibert, L. D. Lise, "Adjuvants: current status, clinical perspectives and future prospects," *Immunology Today* 14 (1993): 281–284; R. Bomford, "Aluminum salts: perspectives in their use as adjuvants," *Immunological Adjuvants and Vaccines* (New York: Plenum Press, 1989): 35–41; N. Petrovsky, "Vaccine Adjuvants: Current State and Future Trends" (2004): 488–496; R. K. Gupta et al., "Adjuvants–a balance between toxicity and adjuvanticity," *Vaccine* 11, no. 4 (1993); and N. Petrovsky, J. C. Aguilar, "Vaccine Adjuvants: Current state and future trends," *Immunology and Cell Biology* 82 (2004): 488–496. Research into the risks of vaccines is inadequate, according to two comprehensive reports on vaccines by the US Institute of Medicine www.iom.edu in 1991 and 1994. The emerging nightmare scenario of inverse or reverse anaphylaxis describes an anaphylactic reaction not to an allergen or antigen (virus, bacteria) but to an antibody.

67. R. Edelman, "Vaccine adjuvants," *Reviews of Infectious Diseases* 2, no. 3 (1980): 370–383.

68. Petrovsky, "Vaccine Adjuvants," 488.

69. D. E. S. Stewart-Tull, "Harmful and Beneficial Activities of Immunological Adjuvants," *Vaccine Adjuvants: Preparation Methods and Research Protocols* (Humana Press, New Jersey, 2000): 30.

70. J. A. Reynolds et al., "Adjuvant activity of a novel metabolizable lipid emulsion with inactivated viral vaccines," *Infection and Immunity* 28, no. 3 (June 1980): 937–943.

71. www.patentstorm.us/patents/6299884/description.html; www.wipo.int/pctdb/ en/wo.jsp?IA=WO2003018051&DISPLAY=DESC; U.S. Patent 5679356; United States Patent 7361352; P. Gecher (ed.), *Encyclopedia of Emulsion Technology: Applications* (Marcel Dekker, 1985) 191; and A. C. Allison, N. E. Byars, "Immunologic adjuvants: General properties, and side-effects," *Molecular Immunology* 28, no. 3 (March 1991): 279–84.

72. K. Pollard, *Autoantibodies and Autoimmunity* (Wiley-VDH, 2006): 54.

73. Stewart-Tull, "Harmful and Beneficial Activities of Immunological Adjuvants," 29.

74. Val Brickates Kennedy, "BioSante: Promise for bird-flu drug," *MarketWatch* (April 24, 2006).

75. M. Khodoun et al., "Peanuts can contribute to anaphylactic shock by activating complement," *J Allergy Clin Immunol* 123, no. 2 (Feb. 2009): 333–351.

76. S. J. Maleki et al., "Structure of the Major Peanut Allergen Ara h 1 May Protect IgE-Binding Epitopes from Degradation," *J. Immunol.* 1, no. 164 (11 (June 2000): 5844–9.

77. Wendy Harris, "Abnormal Response to Normal Things," *Professionally Speaking Magazine, Ontario College of Teachers* (Toronto, Sept. 2000).

78. Institute of Medicine, Committee on Issues and Priorities for New Vaccine Development, *Vaccine Supply and Innovation* (Washington, DC, National Academy Press, 1985): 10.

79. "Vaccination Litigation," *Trial Lawyers Inc., Health Care* (2005). www.triallawyersinc.com/healthcare/hc04.html#notes.

80. Regarding the 1976 "pandemic" see A. M. Silverstein, *Pure Politics and Impure Science* (Johns Hopkins U. Press, 1981). See also A. D. Langmuir et al., "An epidemiologic and Clinical Evaluation of Guillain-Barré Syndrome Reported in Association with the Administration of Swine Influenza Vaccines," *American Journal of Epidemiology* 119, no. 6 (1984): 841–79.

81. *Vaccination Litigation*, Trial Lawyers, Inc. (2005) cites E. W. Kitch, *Vaccines and Product Liability: A Case of Contagious Litigation*, Regulation (May/June 1985): 13.

82. Ibid. "Statement of Robert B. Johnson, president, Lederle Laboratories Division, American Cyanamid, House Subcommittee on Health and the Environment," *Vaccine Injury Compensation* (Sept. 10, 1984).

83. Galambos, *Networks of Innovation*, 148.

84. Institute of Medicine, Committee on Issues and Priorities for New Vaccine Development, *Vaccine Supply and Innovation* (Washington DC, National Academy Press, 1985). The National Institute of Allergy and Infectious Diseases (NIAID, part of the National Institute of Health) proposed an acceleration program for new vaccines. The Dept. of Health and Human Services would conduct the program. The steering committee of the Department of Health and Human Services launched a study of the problem. Three studies emerged in 1985 produced by the Institute of Medicine.

85. Eligible claims are for reactions must have lasted more than six months after the vaccine was given, resulted in hospital stay, surgery or death. The Vaccine Adverse Event Reporting System cosponsored by the FDA and the CDC established in 1990 is not linked to the VICP.

86. Galambos, *Networks of Innovation*, 178.

87. Statistical Abstracts of the United States, *Percent of Children Immunized Against Specific Diseases, by Age Group: 1980 to 1985*. See also F. T. Cutts et al., "Causes of Low Preschool Immunization Coverage in the United States," *Annual Review of Public Health* 13 (May 1992): 385–398.

88. "Improving the Chances of Survival," *The World Health Report, Chapter 6* (WHO, 2005) www.who.int/whr/2005/chapter6/en/index1.html.

89. IOM, *The Children's Vaccine Initiative: achieving the Vision* (Washington, The National Academies Press, 1993).

90. Institute of Medicine, "Committee on Issues and Priorities for New Vaccine Development," *New Vaccine Development: Establishing Priorities 1* (Washington DC, 1985).

91. Galambos, *Networks of Innovation* 177; and US patent application 06/395743 filed Jan. 6, 1982.

92. A. L. Smith, "Antibiotics and Invasive Haemophilus Influenzae," *New England Journal of Medicine* 294, no. 24 (1976): 1329–31.

93. E. O. Mason et al., "Serotype and ampicillin susceptibility of Haemophilus Influenzae causing system infections in children: 3 years of experience," *Journal of Clinical Microbiology* 15, no. 4 (April 1982): 543–546.

94. www.merck.com/product/usa/pi_circulars/p/pedvax_hib/pedvax_pi.pdf.

95. K. C. Schoendort, "National trends in Haemophilus influenzae meningitis mortality and hospitalization among children, 1980 through 1991," *Pediatrics* 93, no. 4 (April 1994): 663–8.

96. The license was in part based on a clinical trial in North Carolina (1977) that involved 16,000 children aged two months to five years. In another Finnish trial 48,977 children three months to five years were injected with the vaccine. Follow-up studies indicated that it was ineffective and had resulted in adverse reactions. It was also noted that it actually increased incidence of the disease right after immunization, in less than seven days.

97. K. R. Stratton et al., (eds.) IOM, "Haemophilus influenzae Type b Vaccines, Background and History," *Adverse Events Associated with Childhood Vaccines* (Washington, National Academies Press, 1994): 236.

98. D. Goldblatt, "Recent developments in bacterial conjugate vaccines," *Journal of Medical Microbiology* 47 (1998): 563–7.

99. R. S. Daum et al., "Decline in serum antibody to the capsule of Haemophilus influenzae type b in the immediate postimmunization period," *J Pediatr* 114 (1989): 742–747.

100. K. R. Stratton et al., (eds.) IOM, "Causality and Evidence," 238.

101. Ibid., 237.

102. FDA summary for Basis of Approval for ActHIB has important information blacked out including induction of higher levels of Ig_ relative to Ig_ www.fda.

gov/downloads/BiologicsBloodVaccines/Vaccines/ApprovedProducts/UCM109864.pdf.

103. Ibid., 237.

104. Ibid.,

105. Viera Scheibner, *Vaccination* (Australia, McPherson's, 1993): 130.

106. Julie Milstien, B. Candries, "Economics of vaccine development and implementation: changes over he past 20 years" (Geneva, WHO, 1998).

107. G. Rothrock et al., "Haemophilus influenzae Invasive Disease Among Children Aged <5 Years—California, 1990–1996," *JAMA* 280 (1998): 1130–1131.

108. "Current Trends Vaccination Coverage of 2-Year-Old Children—United States, 1993," *Morbidity and Mortality Weekly Report (MMWR), CDC* 43, no. 39 (Oct. 7, 1994): 705–709. Vaccination coverage increased for three vaccines from 1992 to 1993: for three or more doses of Hib, from 28.0% to 49.9%; for three or more doses of poliomyelitis vaccine, from 72.4% to 78.4%; and for three or more doses of DPT/ diphtheria and tetanus toxoids (DT), from 83.0% to 87.2%. Coverage with measles-containing vaccine decreased from 82.5% to 80.8%. Among 19-35-month-olds, 12.7% had received three or more doses of Hep B. From 1992 to 1993, the proportion of children who had received a combined series of four or more doses of DPT/DT, three or more doses of polio vaccine, and one dose of MMR increased from 55.3% to 64.8%, primarily because of increased coverage with the fourth DPT/DT dose (from 59.0% to 71.1%). At the start of 1994, Hib coverage was a record high of 70.6% and hepatitis B was at 25.5%.

109. *Disease prevention through vaccine development and immunization, The U.S. National Vaccine Plan—1994*, Dept. of Health and Human Services, Public Health Service, National Vaccine Program Office (1994).

110. IOM, *Calling the Shots: Immunization Finance Policies and Practices* (Washington, National Academy Press, 2000): 252.

111. Gary Walsh, *Biopharmaceuticals* (John Wiley and Sons, 2003).

112. "Changes to the Australian Standard Vaccination Schedule (1992–2005)," *Vaccine Preventable Diseases and Vaccination Coverage in Australia, 2003 to 2005*, Appendix 4, Department of Health and Ageing, Australian Government. www. health.gov.au.

113. D. M. Salisbury et al., "Vaccine programmes and policies," *British Medical Bulletin* 62 (2002): 201–211. http://bmb.oxfordjournals.org/cgi/content/full/62/1/201.

114. www.healthheritageresearch.com/Pertussis/Pertussis-Vaccine-History-CAN-ex-ho.pdf.

115. "Supplementary statement on newly licensed Haemophilus influenzae type B (Hib) conjugate vaccines in combination with other vaccines recommended for infants," Health Canada (1994). http:// pentaproject.net

116. "Acellular pertussis combined with diphtheria and tetanus toxoids for adolescents and adults," Dept. of Pediatrics, University of Saskatchewan, Saskatoon, SK (Feb. 5, 2004). www.medicine.usask.ca/pediatrics/services/childhood-immunization-schedule-1/pertussis.pdf.

117. Advisory Committee on Immunization Practices, "Combined vaccines for childhood immunization," *Morbidity and Mortality Weekly Report (MMWR)CDC* 48, RR05 (May 14, 1999): 1–15.

118. M. J. Corbel, "Control testing of combined vaccines: A consideration of potential problems and approaches," *Biologicals* 22 (1994): 353–60; J. Eskola et al., "Randomized trial of the effect of co-administration with acellular pertussis DPT vaccine on immunogenicity of Haemophilus influenzae type b conjugate vaccine," *Lancet* 348 (1996): 1688–92; P. A. Di Sant-Agnese, "Combined immunization against diphtheria, tetanus and pertussis in newborn infants," *Pediatrics* 3, no. 3 (March 1949): 333–344; and M. A. Valdes-Dapena, "Sudden and unexpected death in infancy: a review of the world literature 1954–1966," *Pediatrics* 39, no. 1 (Jan. 1967): 123–138. This article reviewed the issue sudden infant death syndrome, SIDS. Commenting on the up to 25,000 infant deaths each year, the author professed to be "woefully ignorant." A connection was soon made between these deaths and vaccination: W. C. Torch, "Diptheria-pertussis-tetanus (DPT) immunization: A potential cause of the sudden infant death syndrome (SIDS). *Neurology* 32, no. 4 (1982): 2. In the mid-1970s Japan raised their vaccination age from two months to two years resulting in a significant drop in incidence of SIDS.

119. R. Dagan, "Reduced response to multiple vaccines sharing common protein epitopes that are administered simultaneously to infants," *Infect Immun* 66, no. 5 (May 1998): 2093–8.

120. ACW Lee et al. "Vitamin K deficiency bleeding revisited," *Hong Kong Journal of Paediatrics* 7, no. 3 (2002): 157–161.

121. JH Tripp, "The vitamin K debacle," *Archives of Disease in Childhood* 79 (1998): 295–299.

122. P. M. Loughnan, P. N. McDougall, "Does intramuscular vitamin K1 act as an unintended depot preparation? *J Paediatr Child Health* 32, no. 3 (1996): 251–4.

123. Matthew J. Hills and Harry Beevers, "An antibody to the castor bean glyoxysmomal lipase (62 kD) also binds to a 62 kD protein in extracts from many young oilseed plants," *Plant Physiol* 85 (1987): 1084–1088.

124. www.merckmanuals.com/professional/print/lexicomp/phytonadione.html; and http://dailymed.nlm.nih.gov/dailymed/fda/fdaDrugXsl.cfm?id= 1448& type=display.

125. H. A. Sampson, "Peanut Allergy," *The New England Journal of Medicine* 346 (2002): 1294–1299.

126. A. M. Barnam, S. L. Lukacs, "Food Allergy Among U.S. Children: Trends in Prevalence and Hospitalizations," *National Centre for Health Statistics, CDC* (Oct. 22, 2008). This trend has continued. Four in every one hundred U.S. children has severe food allergy.

127. S. Allan Bock et al., "Fatalities due to anaphylactic reactions to food," *Journal of Allergy and Clinical Immun* 107, no. 1 (Jan. 2001): 191–93.

128. S. H. Sicherer et al., "Prevalence of peanut and tree nut allergy in the United States determined by means of a random digit dial telephone survey: a 5-year follow up study," *JACI* 112, no. 6 (Dec. 2003): 1203–1207.

129. S. Sicherer et al., "U.S. prevalence of self-reported peanut, tree nut, and sesame allergy: 11-year follow-up," *The Journal of Allergy and Clinical Immunology* 125, no. 6 (June 2010): 1322–1326.

CHAPTER 6: ABSORBING THE COSTS

1. A. W. Taylor-Robinson, "Multiple vaccination effects on atopy," *Allergy* 54 (1999): 398–399.

2. www.cdc.gov/vaccines/pubs/pinkbook/downloads/appendices/B/excipient-table-2.pdf.

3. R. K. Gupta, "Adjuvants, a balance between toxicity and adjuvanticity," *Vaccine* 11, no. 3 (Jan. 1993): 293–306; and R. K. Gupta, G. R. Siber, "Adjuvants for human vaccines—current status, problems and future prospects," *Vaccine* 13, no. 14 (1995): 1263–1276.

4. N. Petrovsky et al., "New-Age Vaccine Adjuvants: Friend or Foe?" *Biopharm International* (August 2, 2007): 6. http://biopharminternational.findpharma.com.

5. D. A. Salmon et al., "Enhancing public confidence in vaccines through independent oversight of postlicensure vaccine safety," *American Journal of Public Health* 94, no. 6 (June 2004): 947–950.

6. P. H. Dennehy, "Active Immunization in the United States: Developments over the Past Decade," *Clin Microbiol Rev* 14, no. 4 (Oct. 2001): 872–908. http://ukpmc.ac.uk/articlerender.cgi?artid=127650; and A. W. Taylor-Robinson, , "Multiple vaccination effects on atopy" (1999).

7. K. Stratton et al., IOM, *Immunization Safety Review: Multiple immunizations and immune dysfunction* (Washington, National Academy Press, 2002): 36.

8. Various, "Workshop on Aluminum in Vaccines", *Transcript, Dept. of Health and Human Services, National Vaccine Program Office and jointly sponsored by Task Force for Child Survival and Development Transcript of meeting held at the Caribe Hilton International Hotel, San Juan, Puerto Rico* 2 (May 11, 2000): 105. This

meeting was attended by representative experts from the WHO, industry, government, academia, and interested individuals.

9. Ibid., 78.

10. Ibid., 191.

11. Stanley Hem, "Absorption and Elimination of Aluminum-containing adjuvants," from "Workshop on Aluminum in Vaccines" (2000).

12. T.L. Vasselev, "Aluminium phosphate but not calcium phosphate stimulates the specific IgE response in guinea pigs to tetanus toxoid," *Allergy*, Vol. 33, No. 3 (June, 1978): 155-9.

13. F. Andre et al., "Gelatin prepared from tuna skin: a risk factor for fish allergy or sensitization?" *Immunology* 130, no. 1 (2003).

14. T. Nakayama, T. Kumagai, "Gelatin Allergy," *Pediatrics* 113, no. 1 (Jan. 2004): 170–171; T. Nakayama et al., "A clinical analysis of gelatin allergy and determination of its causal relationship to the previous administration of gelatin-containing acellular pertussis vaccine combined with diphtheria and tetanus toxoids," *J Allergy Clin Immunol* 103, no. 1 (1999): 321–5; R. Wahl, D. Kleinhans, "IgE-mediated allergic reactions to fruit gums and investigation of cross-reactivity between gelatine and modified gelatine-containing products," *Clin Exp Allergy* 19, no. 1 (1989): 77–80; M. Sakaguchi et al., "Food allergy to gelatin in children with systemic immediate-type reactions, including anaphylaxis, to vaccine," *J Allergy Clin Immunol* 98, no. 1 (1996): 1058–61; J. M. Kelso et al., "Anaphylaxis to measles, mumps, and rubella vaccine mediated by IgE to gelatin," *J Allergy Clin Immunol* 91, no. 4 (1993): 867–72; and S. Singer S et al., "Urticaria following varicella vaccine associated with gelatin allergy," *Vaccine* 17, no. 4 (1999): 3279.

15. T. Nakayama, C. Aizawa, "Change in gelatin content of vaccines associated with reduction in reports of allergic reactions," *J Allergy Clin Immunol.* 106 (2000): 591–592.

16. V. Pool et al., "Prevalence of Anti-gelatin IgE antibodies in people with anaphylaxis after measles-mump-rubella vaccine in the United States," *Pediatrics,* 110, 6 (Dec. 2002): e71; and A. Patja et al., "Allergic Reaction to Measles-Mumps-Rubella Vaccination," *Pediatrics* 107, no. 2 (Feb. 2001): e27.

17. V. Dixon et al., "Did you know this medicine has peanut butter in it doctor?" *Archives of Disease in Childhood* 92, no. 7 (July 2007): 654.

18. L. Heller, "Peanut oil production doubles with new U.S. Golden Peanut refiner," *Food Navigator USA, Financial & Industry* (Jan. 17, 2007). www.foodnavigator-usa.com/Financial-Industry/Peanut-oil-production-doubles-with-new-U.S.-Golden-Peanut-refinery.

19. D. A. Moneret-Vautrin et al., "Risks of milk formulas containing peanut oil contaminated with peanut allergens in infants with atopic dermatitis," *Pediatric Allergy*

and Immunology 5, no. 3 (Dec. 1993): 184–188; and A. Cantani, "Anaphylaxis from peanut oil in infant feedings and medications," *European Review of Medical and Pharmacological Sciences* 2 (1998): 203–206.

20. A. Olszewski et al., "Isolation and characterization of proteic allergens in refined peanut oil," *Clin Exp Allergy* 28, no. 7 (July 1998): 850–9; and Threshold Working Group, "Approaches to Establish Thresholds for Major Food Allergens and for Gluten in Food," *Food Allergens Labeling*, U.S. Food and Drug Administration (March 2006).

21. "Opinion of the Scientific Panel on Dietetic Products, Nutrition and Allergies on a request from the Commission related to a notification fro FEDIOL and IMACE on fully refined peanut oil and fat pursuant to Article 6, paragraph 11 of Directive 2000/13/EC," *The European Food Safety Authority (EFSA) Journal* 133 (Oct. 19, 2004): 1–9.

22. J. B. Greig & Joint FAO/WHO Expert Committee on Food Additives, "Potential allergenicity of refined food products, peanut oils and soya bean oils," *WHO Food Additive Series, International Program on Chemical Safety* 44 (2000): 8. www.inchem.org/documents/jecfa/jecmono/v44jec11.htm.

23. "Listing of Food Additive Status," *Food Additives*, U.S. Food and Drug Administration (March 2009); and Threshold Working Group, "Approaches to Establish Thresholds for Major Food Allergens and for Gluten in Food," *Food Allergens Labeling*, US Food and Drug Administration (March 2006).

24. "Guidelines, Medicinal products for human use, safety, environment and information, Excipients in the label and package leaflet of medicinal products for human use," *European Commission* 3B (Brussels, July 2003): 5. www.emea.europa.eu/pdfs/human/productinfo/3bc7a_200307en.pdf.

25. George Wade, EMEA, "Query Response: Arachis Oil: Inquiry No. 11–273," November 20, 2009. This is an email query response.

26. J. Swarbrick, J. C. Boylan (eds.), *Encyclopedia of pharmaceutical technology* 19 (Basel, Marcel Dekker, 2000): 290.

27. I. N. Glaspole et al., "Anaphylaxis to lemon soap: citrus seed and peanut allergen cross-reactivity," *Ann Allergy Asthma Immunol* 98, no. 3 (March 2007): 286–9.

28. R. Ellis, D. Granoff (ed), *Development and clinical uses of haemophilus b conjugate vaccines* (New York, Marcel Dekker, 1994): 120.

29. J. W. Coleman, M. Blanca, "Mechanisms of drug allergy," *Immunology Today* 19, no. 5 (May 1998): 196–198; A. Cantani, *Pediatric allergy, asthma and immunology* (Germany, Springer, 2008)1150; and A. L. Schocket (ed.), *Clinical management of uticaria and anaphylaxis* (U.S., Marcel Dekker Inc., 1993): 120.

30. M. Frieri, B. Kettelhut (eds.), *Food Hypersensitivity and adverse reactions: A practical guide for diagnosis Clinical Allergy and Immunology* (CRC Press, 1999): 84; and

S. D. Kelleher et al. "Functional Chicken Muslcle Protein Isolates . . ." *53rd Annual Reciprocal Meat Conference, American Meat Science Association* (2000). www. meatscience.org. Beef serum albumin and muscle protein (BSA and BGG) has a molecular weight of between 17 and 66 kDa; albumin in egg 45 kDa.

31.   P. A. Gulig, E. J. Hansen, "Coprecipitation of lipopolysaccharide and the 39,000-molecular-weight major outer membrane protein of Haemophilus influenzae type by by lipopolysaccharide-directed monoclonal antibody," *Infection and Immunity* 49, no. 3 (Sept. 1985): 819–827.

32.   A. Kimura et al., "A minor high-molecular-weight outer membrane protein of Haemophilus influenzae type by is a protective antigen," *Infect Immun* 47, no. 1 (Jan. 1985): 253–259.

33.   Leon S. Kind, L. Roesner, "Enhanced susceptibility of pertussis inoculated mice to pollen extract," *Proc Soc Exp Biol Med.* 100, no. 4 (April 1959): 808–10.

34.   C. Chang, R. Y. Gottshall, "Sensitization to ragweed pollen in Bordetella pertussis-infected or vaccine-injected mice," *Journal of Allergy and Clinical Immunology* 54, no. 1 (July 1974): 20–24.

35.   R. Fischer et al., "Oral and nasal sensitization promote distinct immune responses and reactivity in a mouse model of peanut allergy," *American Journal of Pathology* 167 (2005): 1621–1630; and F. van Wijk et al., "The CD28/CTLA-4-B7 signaling pathway is involved in both allergic sensitization and tolerance induction to orally administered peanut proteins," *The Journal of Immunology* 178 (2007): 6894–6900.

36.   A. van den Biggelaar et al., "Neonatal pneumococcal conjugate vaccine immunization primes T cells for preferential Th2 cytokine expression: a randomized controlled trial in Papua New Guinea," *Vaccine* 27, no. 9 (Feb. 2009): 1340–1347; and D. C. Wilson et al., "The Window of opportunity: pre-pregnancy to 24 months of age, induction of antigen-specific immunity in human neonates and infants," *Nestle Nutrition Workshop, Senior Pediatric Program* 61 (2008): 183–95.

37.   M. R. Nelson et al., Anaphylaxis complicating routine childhood immunization: hemophilus influenza b conjugated vaccine," *Pediatric Asthma, Allergy & Immunology* 14, no. 4 (Dec. 2000): 315–321.

38.   R. Schneerson et al., "Preparation, characterization, and immunogenicity of haemophilus influenzae type b polysaccharide-protein conjugates," *Journal of Experimental Medicine* 152 (1980): 361–375.

39.   A. Schuster et al. "Does pertussis infection induce manifestation of allergy?" *Journal of Molecular Medicine* 71, no. 3 (March 1992): 208–213; A. Dannemann et al., "Specific IgE and IgG4 immune respones to tetanus and diphtheria toxoid in atopic and non-atopic children during the first two years of life," *International Archives of Allergy and Immunology* 111, no. 3 (1996): 262–267; J. Nagel et al., "IgE synthesis in man, development of specific IgE antibodies after immunization with

tetanus-diphtheria (Td) toxoids," *J Immunol* 118, no. 1 (Jan. 1977): 334–41; A. Mark et al., "Immuoglobulin E respones to diphtheria and tetanus toxoids after booster with aluminum absorbed and fluid DT-vaccines," *Vaccine* 13, no. 7 (May 1995): 669–73; D. G. Marsh, M. N. Blumenthal," *Genetic and Environmental Factors in Clinical Allergy*, (University of Minnesota Press, 1990): 92; U. Kosecka et al. "Pertussis adjuvant prolongs intestinal hypersensitivity," *Int Arch Allergy Immunol* 119, no. 3 (July 1999): 205–11; M. Flora Martin-Munoz, "Anaphylactic reaction to diphtheria-tetanus vaccine in a child: specific IgE IgG determinations and cross-reactivity studies," *Vaccine* 20, no. 27–28 (Sept. 2002): 3409–3412; C. Mayorga et al., "Immediate allergy to tetanus toxoid vaccine: determination of immunoglobu-lin E and immunoglobulin G antibodies to allergenic proteins," *Ann Allergy Asthma Immunol.* 90, no. 2 (Feb. 2003): 238–43; B. Bellioni Businco et al., "Allergy to tetanus toxoid vaccine," *Allergy* 56, no. 7 (2001): 701–2; and S. Hadenskog, "Immunoglobulin E Response to Pertussis Toxin in Whooping Cough and after Immunization with a Whole-Cell and an Acellular Pertussis Vaccine," *Int Arch Allergy and Immunology* 89 (1989):156–161.

40. Kosecka, "Pertussis adjuvant prolongs intestinal hypersensitivity" (1999).

41. Xiu-Min Li et al., "Engineered Recombinant peanut protein and heat—killed Listeria monocytogenes co-administration protects against peanut-induced ana-phylaxis," *The Journal of Immunology* 170 (2003): 3289–3295.

42. N. O. Eghafona, "Immune responses following cocktails of inactivated measles vaccine and *Arachis hypogaea* L. (ground nut) or *Cocos nucifera* L. (coconut) oils adjuvant," *Vaccine* 17–18, no. 14 (Dec. 1996): 1703–6.

43. F. Audibert, L. Chedid, "Adjuvant disease induced by mycobacteria, determinants of arthritogenicity," *Agents Actions* 1–3, no. 6 (Feb. 1976): 75–85; and Xiu-min Li et al., "Strain-dependent induction of allergic sensitization caused by peanut allergen DNA immunization in mice," *The Journal of Immunology* 162 (1999): 3045–3052.

44. K. Redhead et al., "Combination of DPT and Haemophilus influenzae type b con-jugate vaccines can affect laboratory evaluation of potency and immunogenicity," *Biologicals* 22, no. 4 (Dec. 1994): 339–45.

45. Petrovsky, "Vaccine Adjuvants: Current State and Future Trends,"(2004): 488.

46. D. E. S. Stewart-Tull, "Harmful and Beneficial Activities of Immunological Adjuvants," *Vaccine Adjuvants: Preparation Methods and Research Protocols* (Humana Press, New Jersey, 2000): 30.

47. Y. S. Lee et al., "Invasive Haemophilus influenzae type b infections in Singapore children: a hospital-based study," *Journal of Paediatrics and Child Health* 36, no. 2 (2000): 125–127.

48. F. S. Lim et al., "Primary vaccination of infants against hepatitis B can be completed using a combined hexavalent diphtheria-tetanus-acellular pertussis-hepatitis

B-inactivated poliomyelitis-Haemophilus influenzae type B vaccine," *Ann Acad Med Singapore* 36, no. 10 (Oct. 2007): 801–6.

49.   D. J. Hill et al., "The frequency of food allergy in Australia and Asia," *Environmental Toxicology and Pharmacology* 4, no. 1–2 (Nov. 1997): 101–110; and L. Shek Pei-Chi, Asst. Prof. Dept. of Pediatrics, National University of Singapore, "Food Allergy in Children" (Jan. 2005). This article is online at: www.med.nus.edu.sg/paed/academic/AP_food_allergy.htm.

50.   C. Crooks et al., "The changing epidemiology of food allergy, implications for New Zealand," *The New Zealand Medical Journal* 121, no. 1271 (April 4, 2008).

51.   Malaria Vaccine, Decision-Making Framework, "Overview of National Immunization Program in Ghana," undated. Online at www.malvacdecsion.net/www.malvacdecision.net/pdfs/Overview%20of%20Immunization%20in%20Ghana%20512-06.pdf. Despite the documented sensitivity to peanut, these children were not actively reactive to the food. An important element in this case appeared to have been the helminths. As discussed in the helminth hypothesis, these intestinal worms render those infected hyporeactive. No one knows at what level they confer allergy suppression, but it appeared that helminths were masking the peanut allergy.

52.   E. N. C. Mills et al., "The prevalence, cost and basis of food allergy across Europe," *Allergy* 62, no. 7 (July 2007): 717–722; and http://ec.europa.eu/research/allergy/pdf/workshop/yazdanbakhsh.pdf.

53.   A. E. Platonov et al., "Economic evaluation of Haemophilus influenzae type b vaccination in Moscow, Russian Federation," *Vaccine* 24, no. 13 (March 2006): 2367–2376.

54.   "Incomplete reporting of research in press releases: Et tu, WHO?" *Indian Journal of Medical Research*, 131 (April 2010): 588–589. www.theoneclickgroup.co.uk/news.php?id=4616#newspost.

55.   www.hibaction.org/resources/presentations/TechnicalHibVaccine.ppt.

56.   A. Kemp, "Severe peanut allergy in Australian children," *Medical Journal of Australia* 183, no. 5 (2005): 277; and A. L. Ponsonby, "A prospective study of the association between home gas appliance use during infancy and subsequent dust mite sensitization and lung function in childhood," *Clin Exp Allergy* 31 (2001): 1544–1552.

57.   Linda Smith, "Nut allergies skyrocket," *The Mercury, The Voice of Tasmania* (Feb. 26, 2009).

58.   Ibid.

59.   M. R. Kilmartin et al., "Immunisation of babies, the mothers' perspective," *Australian Family Physician* 27 (Jan. 1998): S11–4.

60. "Changes to the Australian Standard Vaccination Schedule (1992–2005),"
Communicable Diseases Intelligence 31 (June 2007). In 1995 the DPT vaccination
replaced the CDT vaccination (combined diphtheria tetanus) for children prior to
school entry. In 1992, the MMR vaccine was introduced. In 1993, Hib was
introduced. Combined DPTa-hepB-IPV-Hib was introduced in 2001 and DPTa-
IPV-Hib (PRP-T) in Nov. 2005. In 2001, the combined five-in-one vaccine with
Hib was approved for use in Australia. www.health.gov.au/internet/main/publish-
ing.nsf/Content/cda-cdi31suppl.htm~cda-cdi31suppl-apx4.htm; www.health.gov.
au/internet/main/publishing.nsf/Content/cda-cdi28suppl2d.htm;   "Vaccine
Preventable Diseases and Vaccination Coverage in Australia, 2001 to 2002—
Vaccination Coverage," *Communicable Diseases Intelligence* 28, no. 2 (Dec. 2004);
and "Changes to the Australian Standard Vaccination Schedule (1992–2005),
Communicable Diseases Intelligence 31 (June 2007), www.health.gov.au/internet/
main/publishing.nsf/Content/cda-cdi31suppl.htm~cda-cdi31suppl-apx4.htm.

61. "Vaccine Preventable Diseases and Vaccination Coverage in Australia, 2001 to
2002, Vaccination Coverage," *Communicable Diseases Intelligence* 28, no. 2 (Dec.
2004). www.health.gov.au/internet/main/publishing.nsf/Content/cda-cdi28sup-
pl2d.htm.

62. ACT is a self-governing state within New South Wales with the highest density
population and smallest area at 910 square miles. Within it is the national capital
of Canberra.

63. Linda Smith, "Nut allergies skyrocket," 2009.

64. M. Kijakovic et al., "The parent-reported prevalence and management of peanut
and nut allergy in school children in the Australian Capital Territory," *Journal of
Paediatrics and Child Health* 45 (March 2009); R. J. Mullins, "Characteristics of
childhood peanut allergy in the Australian Capital Territory 1995 to 2007," *J
Allergy and Clin Immunol* 123, no. 3 (March 2009): 689–693; and R. J. Mullins,
"Paediatric food allergy trends in a community-based specialist allergy practice,
1995–2006," *Medical Journal of Australia* 186, no. 12 (2007): 618–621. Over twelve
years, Mullins saw the demand for food allergy services increase 400% in his practice for children aged zero to five. Peanut, tree nut, egg and dairy were the common
triggers. Mullins interpreted the dramatic increase in hospital admissions for anaphylaxis in Australia at twice that described in U.K. studies as evidence of a food
allergy "epidemic."

65. "Health Status: Protecting the health of our children," *Australian Social Trends,
Australian Bureau of Statistics* 41020 (June 1997). www.abs.gov.au.

66. H. A. Sampson, "Peanut Allergy," *The New England Journal of Medicine* 346 (2002):
1294–1299.

67. ACW Lee et al. "Vitamin K deficiency bleeding revisited," *HK J Paediatr* 7, no. 3 (2002): 157–161.

68. J. K. Aronson, *Meyler's Side Effects of Cardiovascular Drugs* (Elsevier, 2004): 508.

69. JH Tripp, "The vitamin K debacle," *Archives of Disease in Childhood* 79 (1998): 295–299.

70. Matthew J. Hills, Harry Beevers, "An antibody to the castor bean glyoxysmomal lipase (62 kD) also binds to a 62 kD protein in extracts from many young oilseed plants," *Plant Physiol* 85 (1987): 1084–1088.

71. P. M. Loughnan, P. N. McDougall, "Does intramuscular vitamin K1 act as an unintended depot preparation?" *J Paediatr Child Health* 32, no. 3 (1996): 251–4.

72. www.merckmanuals.com/professional/print/lexicomp/phytonadione.html; and http://dailymed.nlm.nih.gov/dailymed/fda/fdaDrugXsl.cfm?id= 1448& type= display.

73. Profet, "The Function of Allergy," 36.

74. K. Bock, *Healing the New Childhood Epidemics*, 19.

75. Ibid.

76. T. D. Green, "Clinical Characteristics of Peanut-Allergic Children: Recent Changes," *Pediatrics* 120, no. 6 (Dec. 2007): 1304–1310; S. H. Sicherer et al., "Clinical features of acute allergic reactions to peanut and tree nuts in children," *Pediatrics* 102, no. 1 (1998): e6; T. K. Vander Leek et al., "The natural history of peanut allergy in young children and its association with serum peanut-specific IgE," *J Pediatr* 137 (2000): 749–755; H. S. Skolnik et al., "The natural history of peanut allergy," *J. Allergy Clin Immunol* 107 (2001): 367–374; and Mullins, "Paediatric food allergy trends in a community-based specialist allergy practice, 1995–2006," *Medical Journal of Australia*, 186, 12 (2007): 618–621.

77. S. Sicherer et al., "Prevalence of peanut and tree nut allergy in the United States determined by means of a random digit dial telephone survey: a 5 year follow up study," *Journal of Allergy and Clin Immunol* 112 (2003): 1203–1207.

78. S. Cave, "Testimony," Committee on Government Reform, U.S. House of Representatives (July 18, 2000). www.healing-arts.org/children/autismandmercurytestimony.htm.

CHAPTER 7: RATIONALIZATIONS

1. N. Petrovsky et al., "New-Age Vaccine Adjuvants: Friend or Foe?" *Biopharm International* (August 2, 2007): 6. http://biopharminternational.findpharma.com.

2. T. Nakayama, T. Kumagai, "Gelatin Allergy," *Pediatrics* 113, no. 1; (Jan. 2004): 170–171.

3. Stuart Anderson, *Making Medicines: a brief history of pharmacy and pharmaceuticals* (Pharmaceutical Press, 2005): 156.

4. A. W. Taylor-Robinson, "Multiple vaccination effects on atopy," *Allergy* 54 (1999): 398–399.

5. Charles Richet, *The Nobel Prize in Physiology or Medicine 1913, Nobel Lecture* (Dec. 11, 1913). http://nobelprize.org/nobel_prizes/medicine/laureates/1913/richet-lecture.html.

6. C. Anandan, A. Sheikh, "Preventing development of allergic disorders in children," *BMJ* 333 (2006): 485.

7. *Scientific Review of Vaccine Safety Datalink Information*, Simpsonwood Retreat Center, Norcross Georgia (June 7–8, 2000). In attendance at this meeting called by the Centers for Disease Control were the CDC's Advisory Committee on Immunization Practices (ACIP), American Academy of Pediatrics (AAP) and forty-eight other well-regarded institutions as well as members from GlaxoSmithKline, Merck, Wyeth, and Aventis Pasteur. Both transcript and report are available at www.autismhelpforyou.com. The report and transcript are discussed in Robert F. Kennedy Jr., "Deadly Immunity," *Salon.com* (June 16, 2005).

8. "The Man Behind the Vaccine Mystery," *CBS Evening News* (Dec. 12, 2002). www.cbsnews.com.

9. Various, *Scientific Review of Vaccine Safety Datalink Information*, Transcript of Meeting held at the Simpsonwood Retreat Center, Norcross Georgia (June 7–8, 2000): 248.

10. "Study Autism prevalence still up after thimerosal removed from vaccines, New genetic link found," *American Academy of Family Physicians* (Jan. 16, 2008). www. aafp.org. Also, Anon, "Influenza vaccination coverage among pregnant women, United States, 2012-13 influenza season," *Morbidity and Mortality Weekly Report* (MMWR) Sept. 27, 2013. http://www.cdc.gov/mmwr/preview/mmwrhtml/mm6238a3.htm

11. Alice Park, "The Truth About Vaccines," *Time Magazine* (Canadian Edition, June 2, 2008): 34.

12. *Tim Vawter v Federal government*, presented to U.S. DNY on July 31, 2009. www. safetylawsuits.com/prelim-injunction.html. The injunction was filed simultaneously with WHO news that one billion doses of adjuvanted H1N1 swine flu vaccine containing thimerosal had been sold to Western countries. "Canada to order 50.4 million H1N1 vaccine doses," *CBC News*, Aug. 6, 2009. www.cbc.ca/health/story/2009/08/06/swine-flu-vaccine.html. In Canada the government contract for 50.4 million doses costing $40 million was granted to Glaxo SmithKline which uses an "adjuvant advantage."

13. Val Brickates Kennedy, "BioSante: Promise for bird flu drug," *MarketWatch* (April 24, 2006).

14. "Seasonal Influenza: the economics of vaccination," *Center for Prevention and Health Services* (Oct. 2006).

15. C. W. Shepard et al., "Cost-effectiveness of conjugate meningococcal vaccination strategies in the United States," *Pediatrics* 115, no. 5 (May 2005): 1220–1232.

16. Julie Milstien, B. Candries, "Economics of vaccine development and implementation: changes over he past 20 years" (Geneva, WHO, 1998). www.who. int/immunization_supply/introduction/economics_vaccineproduction.pdf.

17. Rep. Henry A. Waxman, "Analysis, pharmaceutical industry profits increase by over $8 billion after Medicare drug plan goes into effect," Report, Rep. Henry A. Waxman, Ranking Minority member, Committee on Government Reform, U.S. House of Representatives, Sept. 2006. http://oversight.house.gov/documents/20060919115623 -70677.pdf.

18. Annys Shin, "Food allergies trigger multibillion-dollar specialty market," *The Washington Post* (Sun., June 8, 2008). Online: www.washingtonpost.com/wp-dyn/content/article/2008/06/07/AR2008060702125.html.

19. James Altucher, "Save the children (and make money)," *Wall Street Journal, Investing* (August 10, 2009). http://online.wsj.com/article/SB12499239038 7319939.html.

20. Dr. Eugene Robin, "Letter to The First International Public Conference on Vaccination", *Mothering* 86 (January/February 1998). Reprinted in www.mothering.com/health/first-international-public-conference-vaccination.

21. National Adult Immunization Plan, National Vaccine Program Office (Feb. 5, 2015) In Canada, few parents in Canada realize that if their child is injured neither doctor nor manufacturer nor government accepts any legal liability. You are on your own.

22. "Supplementary statement on newly licensed Haemophilus influenzae type B (Hib) conjugate vaccines in combination with other vaccines recommended for infants", Canadian Medical Association Journal, 1995 (152) 527-529.

23. "Acellular pertussis combined with diphtheria and tetanus toxoids for adolescents and adults," Dept. of Pediatrics, University of Saskatchewan, SK (Feb. 5, 2004).

CHAPTER 8 THE BUSINESS OF BREATHLESSNESS & OOZING SKIN

1. Samuel Hahnemann, The *Organon of Medicine*, (5th ed., 1833) p. 49-50.

2. Ivan Illich, *Medical Nemesis: The Expropriation of Health* (NY, Pantheon books, 1976) p. 3.

3. Jared Diamond, *Guns, Germs and Steel* (NY, W. Norton & Co., 1997) p. 202.

4. https://www.youtube.com/watch?v=0_o5z_Gq-BU   http://www.petervadasmd.com/mediaappearances.html

5. K.B. Saunders, "Origin of the word 'asthma,'" *Thorax*, No. 48 (1993): 647.

6.	William Cullen, *Synopsia Nosologiae Methodicae*, (Edinburgh, Kincaid & Creech, 1769) from L. Juhlin, "The History of Urticaria and Angioedema," *Forum for Nord Derm Ven*, Vol. 6 (May 2001).

7.	William Cullen, *The Edinburgh Practice of Physic, Surgery, and Midwifery*, Vol. 2 (London, Kearsley, 1803) 389-394. https://books.google.ca/books?id=aegzJMUcP_gC&pg=PA389&dq=william+cullen,+asthma&hl=en&ei=EEvJTd7fHuTl0QGMqPTzBw&sa=X&oi=book_result&ct=result&redir_esc=y#v=onepage&q&f=false

8.	G.M. Beard, *American Nervousness: Its Causes and Consequences* (NY, Putnam's Sons, 1881).

9.	M. Ramachandran et al., "John Bostock's first description of hayfever," *JR Soc Med*. Vol. 104, No. 6 (2011): 237-240.

10.	C.H. Blackley, *Experimental researches on the cause and nature of catarrhus aestivus* (hay-fever or hay-asthma), (London, Balliere, Tindall and Cox, 1873) p. 35.

11.	Gregg Mitman, "Hay Fever Holiday: Health, leisure, and place in Gilded-Age America," *Bull. Hist. Med.*, 77 (2003): 600-635.

12.	"Hay Fever," *White Mountain Echo* (Sept. 13, 1879) p. 1. Quoted in Gregg Mitman, "Hay Fever Holiday: Health, leisure, and place in Gilded-Age America," *Bull. Hist. Med.*, 77 (2003):600-635.

13.	Mark Jackson, "Divine Stramonium": the rise and fall of smoking for asthma," *Med Hist.*, No. 54, Vol. 2 (2010): 171-194. https://www.ncbi.nlm.nih.gov/pmc/articles/PMC2844275/

14.	Gregg Mitman, *Breathing Space: how allergies shape our lives and landscapes* (New Haven, Yale U. Press, 2007) p. 56.

15.	Samuel Hahnemann, *The Organon of Medicine* (1833).

16.	Ibid, p. ix.

17.	From the letters of Charles Darwin in F. Orrego, et al. "Darwin's illness: a final diagnosis," *The Royal Society Journal of the History of Science* (2007).

18.	J. Whorton, *The Arsenic Century: How Victorian Britain was Poisoned at Home, Work and Play* (Oxford U. Press, 2010).

19.	C. Richet, *Thirty Years of Psychical Research Being a Treatise on Metaphysics* (New York, MacMillan Co., 1923).

20.	Ibid, p. 433.

21.	Term coined by Nobel Laureate and chemist Svante Arrhenius in 1904.

22.	Foucault, *Birth of the Clinic* (London, Routledge Classics, 2003) p. 147.

23.	J.M. Igea, "The history of the idea of allergy," *Allergy*, 68 (2013): 966-973.

24.	R. C. Dreyfuss, J.C. Ginsburg, *Intellectual Property at the Edge* (Cambridge University Press, 2014) p. 324. Also, Brian Hoffman, *Adrenaline* (Cambridge, Harvard U. Press, 2013).

25. Parke-Davis & Co. v. H.K. Mulford Co. Circuit Court, S.D. New York, 189, F. 95; 1911 U.S. App. LEXIS 5245, April 28, 1911. http://www.pubpat.org/assets/files/brca/mats/Parke-Davis,%20189%20Fed%2095%20(1911).pdf

26. Mark Jackson, *Asthma* (Oxford Unversity Press, 2009) p. 134.

27. P.W.L. Camps, "A note on the inhalation treatment of asthma," *Guy's Hosp. Rep.*, 79 (1929): 496-8. This from N.Jones, *The Ins and Outs of Breathing* (iUniverse, 2011).

28. https://www.ncbi.nlm.nih.gov/pmc/articles/PMC1760721/ M. Parsons et al., "Histamine and its receptors," *Br J. Pharmacol.*, Vol. 147 (2006): S127-S135.

29. C. Sager, "Geoerge Rieveschl: Benadryl," *Stuff of Genius* (Aug. 14, 2013).

30. D. Abrams, *Ernesto "Che" Guevara* (NYC, Chelsea House, 2010).

31. Anon, "Cuba, Castro's Brain," *Time* (Aug. 8, 1960).

32. J. Casta, *Companero: The Life and Death of Che Guevara* (Vintage, 1998).

33. Ibid, p. 102.

34. M. Jackson, *Asthma*, p. 162

35. Casta, op cit, p. 194.

36. P. Stolley, "Asthma Mortality: Why the United States was spared an epidemic of deaths due to asthma," *American Review of Respiratory Disease*, Vol. 105 (1972): 833. From M. Silverman, P. Lee, Pills, *Profits and Politics* (U. of California Press, 1974).

37. R. Cooke, "The Treatment of Hay Fever by Active Immunization," *Laryngoscope*, Vol. 25, Issue 2 (1915): p. 108. Cooke's work was based on that of French physician Alexandre Besredka. Besredka hypothesized in 1907 that the nervous system was involved in anaphylaxis – he predicted later research in the role of thought/stress and the nervous and immune systems (psycho-neuro-immunology) manifesting in allergy (or the reverse where food allergy impacts the brain).

38. Colin Wilson, "Prevention of Hay Fever by Pollaccine," *J R Army Med Corps*. Vol. 45 (1925): 380-381.

39. Warren T. Vaughan, *Primer of Allergy* (St. Louis, Mosby, 1939) p. 89.

40. A. Sheikh, et al., *Landmark Papers in Allergy* (Oxford, Oxford U. Press, 2013) p. 50.

41. Cooke, et al. "Serological evidence of immunity with coexisting sensitization in type of human allergy (hay fever)", *J Exp Med.*, Vol. 62 (1935): 73-50

42. A. Sheikh, et al., *Landmark Papers in Allergy*, p. 45, 65.

43. R. Suter, "Emergency medicine in the United States," *World J Emerg Med.*, Vol. 3, No. 1 (2012): 5-10.

44. A. de Weck, et al, *Allergic Reactions to Drugs* (Berlin, Springer, 1983) p. 6

45. Jackson, *Asthma*, p. 11.

46. R. Jaslow, "Food allergies cost US $25 billion a year," *CBS News* (Sept. 25, 2013).

47. K. Tunney, "How Many People Use EpiPens in America?" *Bustle* (Aug. 26, 2016).

48.   As already noted, allergy may be defined as an evolved defense against acute toxicity. This book argues that the provocative and toxic nature of vaccination was and is the primary precipitating cause of the current epidemic. That is not to say that there are not other means by which people become anaphylactic. This I have also made clear in this book.

49.   James Altucher "Save the children (and make money)" *The Wall Street Journal* (Aug.10, 2009) online.wsj.com/article SB124992390387319939.html

50.   A. Baltabekova, et al, "Split Core Technology allows efficient production of virus-like particles presenting a receptor-contacting epitope of human IgE," *Molecular Biotech*, Vol. 57 (2015): 746-755.

51.   Vaccines for suppressing IgE mediated allergic disease and methods for using the same US 9408897 B2 granted Aug. 9, 2016.

52.   E. Nigro et al., "Role and redirection of IgE against cancer," *Antibodies*, Vol. 2 (2013): 371-391.

53.   Stacie M. Jones et al. "Epicutaneous immunotherapy for the treatment of peanut allergy in children and young adults." *J. Allergy Clin. Immunol.* (2016)

54.   K. Doheny, "Peanut Allergy Treatment: the earlier in childhood, the better," *Health Day* (Aug. 2016).

55.   J. Stern et al., "Relation between eosinophilic esophagitis and oral immunotherapy for food allergy," *Pediatrics*,Vol. 136 (2015).

56.   W. Dawicki et al., "Therapeutic reversal of food allergen sensitivity by mature retinoic acid-differentiated dendritic cell induction of LAG3+CD49b-Foxp3- regulatory T cells," *JACI* (2016).

57.   XM Li et al, "The Chinese herbal medicine formula FAHF-2 completely blocks anaphylactic reactions in a murine model of peanut allergy," *J Allergy Clin Immunol.* 115 (2005): 171-8.

58.   Michel Foucault, "The Crisis of Medicine or the Crisis of Antimedicine?" *Foucault Studies*, No. 1 (Dec. 2004) p. 5

59.   Gilbert Ryle, *The Concept of Mind* (University of Chicago Press, 1949).

APPENDIX

1.   A.S. Amoah, et al., "Peanut specific IgE antibodies in asymptomatic Ghanaian children possibly caused by carbohydrate determinant cross reactivity," *J Allergy Clin Immunol.*, 132, 3 (2013): 639-647.

2.   D. M. Lewis, General Practitioner, Watford, UK, Letter in response to C. Anandan, A. Sheikh, "Preventing development of allergic disorders in children," *BMJ*, 333 (2006): 485.

3. Daniel Boakye, "Infections and Food Allergy in Africa," Noguchi Memorial Institute for Medical Research http://ec.europa.eu; and B. B. Obeng et al., "Allergic sensitization and reported adverse reactions to food in Ghanaian school children: a nested case-control study," *Journal of Allergy and Clinical Immunology* 123, no. 2 (Feb. 2009): S31.

4. Levin, M.E. et al., "Associations between asthma and bronchial hyper responsiveness with allergy and atopy phenotypes in urban black south African teenagers," *South African Med J*, 101, 7 (2011): 472-476. Also, G. Du Toit et al., "Peanut allergy and peanut-specific IgG4 characteristics among Xhosan children in Cape Town," *J Allergy Clin Immunol* 119, no. 1 (Jan. 2007): S196. Malnourishment of children is a significant problem in Algeria, for example, where fat based spread fortified with nutrients is made from dried lactoserum and peanut butter. Allergic reaction has not been a problem in the settings where the spread has been used by a WHO field trial in Algeria.

5. M. Kijakovic et al., "The parent-reported prevalence and management of peanut and nut allergy in school children in the Australian Capital Territory," *Journal of Paediatrics and Child Health* 45 (March 2009): 3; and R. J. Mullins, "Paediatric food allergy trends in a community-based specialist allergy practice, 1995–2006," *Medical Journal of Australia* 186, no. 12 (2007): 618–621.

6. "Better information urgently needed as childhood peanut allergy rate climbs," *The Australian Society of Clinical Immunology and Allergy* (Feb. 25, 2009). www.allergy.org.au/content/view/360/76/.

7. R. J. Mullins, "Characteristics of childhood peanut allergy in the Australian Capital Territory 1995 to 2007," *J Allergy and Clin Immunol* 123, no. 3 (March 2009): 689–693.

8. Linda Smith, "Nut allergies skyrocket."

9. Osborne, N.J., et al., "Prevalence of challenge proven IgE mediated food allergy using population sample and predetermined challenge criteria in infants," *J Allergy Clin Immunol.*, 127, 3 (2011): 668-76.

10. Linda Smith, "Nut allergies skyrocket," *The Mercury, The Voice of Tasmania* (Feb. 26, 2009).

11. A. Kemp, "Severe peanut allergy in Australian children," *Med J of Australia* 183, no. 5 (2005): 277; and A. L. Ponsonby et al., "A prospective study of the association between home gas appliance use during infancy and subsequent dust mite sensitization and lung function in childhood," *Clin Exp Allergy* 31 (2001): 1544–1552.

12. Soller, L., et al., "Overall prevalence of self-reported food allergy in Canada," *J Allergy Immunol.* (2012).

13. A team from McGill University conducted the first temporal survey of peanut allergy in North America. In 2000/2002, they surveyed 4,339 schoolchildren in

Montreal and found that 1.5% of the children in kindergarten through third grade—between the ages of five and nine—had peanut and/or nut allergies. In a five-year follow-up study they found that prevalence of this allergy had increased to 1.71% in 2005/07. In five years prevalence of peanut allergy in Montreal children had increased 35%. This may hold true for all Canadian children. A survey of anaphylaxis in 2000–01 in Canada indicated that 1.44% of the pediatric population under seventeen years had portable, EpiPen epinephrine dispensed. This was believed to underrepresent teens and reflect an underestimation of true occurrence rate of anaphylaxis. F. Estelle et al., "Allergy Frontiers and Futures," *Allergy Clin Immunol Int* 242, no. 1 (2004); and M. Ben-Shoshan et al., "Is the prevalence of peanut allergy increasing? A five-year follow-up study on the prevalence of peanut allergy in Montreal school children aged 5 to 9 years," *The Journal of Allergy and Clinical Immunology* 121, no. 2; (Feb. 2008): S97.

14. N. E. Eriksson et al., "Self-reported food hypersensitivity in Sweden, Denmark, Estonia, Lithuania and Russia," *J Invest Allergol Clin Immunol* 14 (2004): 70–79.

15. Dubakiene, R. Et al., "Studies on early allergic sensitization in the Lithuanian birth cohort," *The Scientific World Journal* (2012).

16. Fedeorova, O.S., et al., "The prevalence of food allergy to peanut and hazelnut in children in Tomsk Region," *Vopr Pitan.* 83, 1 (2014): 48-54.

17. In France, a 2002 study of children in Toulouse schools found that 6.7% of all children had true food allergies, this compared to the 4.7% of U.S. children. Cow milk, eggs and peanuts were the main foods reported where 8.2% of children of all ages reported having an adverse reaction to peanut. It was unclear as to the exact percentage anaphylactic to peanut. Overall, the rate of peanut sensitization could be between 1.05% and 2.5% of the overall population. Eighteen% of the population of France was under fifteen in 2002 indicating that 0.45% of children were allergic to peanuts. F. Rancé, "Prevalence and main characteristics of schoolchildren diagnosed with food allergies in France," *Clinical and Experimental Allergy* 35, no. 2 (Feb. 2005): 167–172; and M. Morisset et al., "Prevalence of peanut sensitization in a population of 4,137 patients referred to allergologists," *AllergoVigilance Network* (2002). www.cicbaa.com/pages_us/allergovigilance/prevalencepeanut.pdf.

18. A. Mehl et al., "Anaphylactic reactions in children—a questionnaire-based survey in Germany," *Allergy* 60, no. 11 (Nov. 2005):1440–1445.

19. C. Roehr et al., "Food allergy and non-allergic food hypersensitivity in children and adolescents," *Clin Exp Allergy* 34, no. 1 (Oct. 2004): 1534–41.

20. T. F. Leung et al., "Parent-reported adverse food reactions in Hong Kong Chinese preschoolers: epidemiology, clinical spectrum and risk factors," *Pediatric Allergy & Immunology* 20, no. 4 (June 2009): 339–346. About 3,800 children ages two to seven living in Hong Kong were recruited. Parents reported 8.1% adverse food

reactions and doctors confirmed 4.6%. Top 3 causes of AFR were shellfish, egg, peanut (8.1%). AFR is a common atopic disorder in Hong Kong preschool children, and prevalence rates are comparable to Caucasians. Mainland China fewer parent reported AFR in 4%.

21. R. Hatahet et al., "Sensibilisation aux allergens d'arachide chez les nourrissons de moins de quarter mois: à propos de 125 observations," *Rev Fr Allergol Immunol Clin* 34 (1994): 377–81.

22. D. J. Hill et al., "Clinical spectrum of food allergy in children in Australia and South-East Asia: identification and targets for treatment," *Annals of Medicine* 31, no. 4 (Aug. 1999): 272–81. Despite the high rate of peanut consumption it is a are allergen. Allergy to all foods affects 3.4% to 5% of the residents in Beijing, Guangdong, and the Sheng-Li oil fields. Top allergens include fish, shrimp, crab and seaweed. In twenty-nine children aged two to twelve years with diagnosed food allergy in the Chinese population studied, none had signs of clinical allergy to peanut, although 2% of them were skin-test positive to peanut in 1999.

23. T. F. Leung, "Sensitization to common food allergens is a risk factor for asthma in young Chinese children in Hong Kong," *Journal of Asthma* 39, no. 6 (Sept. 2002): 523–9.

24. K., Beyer K et al., "Effects of cooking methods on peanut allergenicity," *J Allergy Clin Immunol* 107, no. 6 (2001): 1077–1081.

25. Mangala M. Pai, Assist. Prof., Centre for Basic Sciences, KMC, Mangalore, Bejai "Peanut allergy-prevention?" *BMJ* (Sept. 2006).

26. Graif, Yael, et al., "Association of food allergy and asthma severity and atopic diseases in Jewish and Arab adolescents," *Acta Paediatri*, 101, 10 (2012): 1083-8.

27. D. Aaronov et al., "Natural history of food allergy in infants and children in Israel," *Ann Allergy Asthma Immunol* 101, 6 (Dec. 2008): 637–40.

28. M. Ebisawa et al., "Food allergy in Japan," *Allergy Clin Immunol Int* 15 (May 2003): 214–7.

29. C.G Mortz et al., "The prevalence of peanut sensitization and the association to pollen sensitization in a cohort of unselected adolescents," *Pediatric Allergy & Immunology* 16, no. 6 (Sept. 2005): 501–506.

30. Ibid.

31. C. Crooks et al., "The changing epidemiology of food allergy, implications for New Zealand," *The New Zealand Medical Journal* 121, no. 1271 (April 4, 2008).

32. D. J. Hill et al., "The frequency of food allergy in Australia and Asia," *Environmental Toxicology and Pharmacology* 4, no. 1–2 (Nov. 1997): 101–110.

33. L. Shek Pei-Chi, L. Shek Pei-Chi, Asst. Prof. Dept. of Pediatrics, National University of Singapore, "Food Allergy in Children" (Jan. 2005).

34. C. Crooks "The changing epidemiology of food allergy, implications for New Zealand."

35. Sweden exhibits a very high prevalence of peanut allergy but Denmark and Norway very low. Per capita consumption of peanut in Sweden is low at 0.8kg per person compared with 2.1 kg in the United States. In a study of children who were tested for IgE antibodies for peanut between January 1994 and 1998, authors found similar course of events for young children under six in the United States. Occurrence of peanut allergy had increased without a country wide increase in consumption. J. Van Odijk et al., "Specific immunoglobulin E antibodies to peanut over time in relation to peanut intake, symptoms and age," *Pediatric Allergy & Immunolog* 15, no. 5 (Oct. 2004): 442–448; and J. Van Odijk et al., "Specific IgE antibodies to peanut in western Sweden—has the occurrence of peanut allergy increased without an increase in consumption?" *Allergy* 56, no. 6 (June 2001): 573–7.

36. Hourihane J, et al. "The impact of government advice to pregnant mothers regarding peanut avoidance on the prevalence of peanut allergy in United Kingdom children at school entry," *J Allergy Clin Immunol.* 119 (2007): 1197–1202; and *British Society for Allergy & Clinical Immunology.* www.bsaci.org.

37. The LEAP study authors have stated that one in seventy U.K. children suffers from peanut allergy and that the vast majority (80%) will have the allergy for life. In a population based study of three-year-olds in the United Kingdom, the prevalence of sensitization to peanuts increased from 1.3 percent to 3.2 percent between 1989 and1995. In 1998, the U.K. Department of Health recommended that mothers from "high-risk" families (those with a history of atopy) avoid eating peanuts during pregnancy and lactation and that they not give their infants peanut products for the first three years of life. Isle of Wight study at the David Hide Asthma and Allergy Research Centre found that the numbers of children who tested positive for peanut tripled between 1989 and 1996: 1.1% of children in 1989 compared to 3.3% in 1996. J. Grundy et al. "Rising prevalence of allergy to peanut in children: data from 2 sequential cohorts," *J Allergy Clin Immunol* 110 (2002): 784–9; J. Grundy, et al., "Peanut allergy in three year old children—a population based study," *J. Allergy Clin Immunol* 107 (2001): S231; and Committee on Toxicity of Chemicals in Food, Consumer Products, and the Environment, *Peanut allergy* (London: Department of Health, 1998): 1–57.

38. Gupta, R.S., et al., "Understanding the prevalence of childhood food allergy in the United States," *Pediatrics* (2011).

39. Sicherer, S., et al. "U.S. Prevalence of Self-Reported Peanut, Tree Nut, and Sesame Allergy: 11-Year Follow-Up," *J Allergy Clin Immunol* 125, no. 6 (June 2010): 1322–1326.

40.   Prevalence of peanut and tree nut allergy in the United States was determined by a telephone survey with a five-year follow-up. A team of researchers found that the rate of peanut/tree nut allergies increased significantly in children but not at all in adults. The number of allergic children had doubled from 0.6% in 1997 to 1.2% in 2002. And one of the most puzzling facts is that 9% of Americans had "serologic evidence" of sensitivity to peanuts according to the CDC's National Health and Nutrition Examination Survey (NHANE III data was collected from 1988 to 1994). S. H. Sicherer et al. "Prevalence of peanut and tree nut allergy in the United States determined by means of a random digit dial telephone survey: a 5-year follow up study," *The Journal of Allergy and Clinical Immunology*, 112, no. 6 (Dec. 2003,): 1203–1207; S. Sicherer et al., "Prevalence of peanut and tree nut allergy in the United States determined by a random digit dial telephone survey," *J of Allergy and Clin Immunology* 103 (1999): 559–62; A. M. Barnum, S. L. Lukacs, "Food allergy among US children: trends in prevalence and hospitalizations," National Center for Health Statistics, CDC (Oct. 22, 2008). In 2003, 4.7% of children less than five years had food allergies and about 6% to 8 percent of children younger than 4. Since 1998, there had been an 18% increase; DeNoon, DJ. "Food allergy in kids up 18%," *MedicineNet.com* (Oct. 22, 2008); Mike Stobbe, "Food allergies increasing in U.S. kids," *SF Gate* (Oct. 22, 2008). The CDC used data from a National Health Interview Survey which sampled 9,500 children in 2007 and the National Hospital Discharge Survey which includes 270,000 inpatient records from five hundred hospitals; Chiu L, "Estimation of the sensitization rate to peanut by prick skin test in the general population: results from the National Health and Nutrition Examination Survey, 1980–1994," *J Allergy Clin Immunol* 107 (2001): S192; and Sicherer, S. et al. "Prevalence of Peanut and Tree Nut Allergy in the US determined by a Random Digit Dial Telephone Survey."

INDEX